"With each page of her amazing book, Arlene Pellicane identifies secrets for growing younger—secrets so obvious, so easy, so much fun to do, readers will wonder why they haven't heard them before. Each page of this must-read book will bring a smile to your face, a fresh attitude to your life, a quickness to your step, and a radiance causing others to ask your secret. Through reading *31 Days to a Younger You*, your life and the lives of those you know and love will be blessed, and honor and glory will come to God who 'fearfully and wonderfully' made you."

—Melvin L. Cheatham, MD,
clinical professor of neurosurgery, UCLA Medical Center,
and member of the board of directors of Samaritan's Purse

"Simple truths are sometimes overlooked or taken for granted. *31 Days to a Younger You* opens your eyes and unplugs your ears to what we all want—a healthier life and more appealing physical features. Reading it called my attention to the choices we have to look younger without the regimen of dieting, surgery, and more. Read this book and be ready to look better, think clearer, love yourself easier, and inspire others by these simple and successful ways to stay younger than you look and feel."

—Dr. Thelma Wells, president,
A Woman of God Ministries

"There is not an aspect of life and living that Arlene Pellicane does not delve into in *31 Days to a Younger You*. This beautiful, savvy young mom shares secrets and wisdom that will woo you to a richer, fuller, happier life—whether you are 16 or 60. Packed with encouragement, advice, and the motivation to embrace it all, this book is worth the read."

—Terry Meeuwsen, cohost, *The 700 Club*

"While women today have more opportunities than ever before, they also face more pressure to look younger and more attractive in order to compete, both in the workplace and in life. Arlene's book is a breath of fresh air for women. With her priorities in order, this active mom and author emphasizes the beauty of the heart without downplaying the importance of physical health and appearance. The simple strategies in her book will make you feel and look younger."

San Diego TV news anchor

"This book had me looking forward to my quiet time in a refreshing new way. It was like taking a daily coffee break with a good friend and chatting about our personal issues with each conversation circling back to the importance of God in our everyday lives. Arlene's delightful sense of humor and warmth come through her writing as she gives tips and tidbits of advice on ways *any* woman can look and feel gorgeous without feeling guilty."

—**Jill Swanson,** image coach,
author of *Simply Beautiful—Inside and Out*

"Arlene Pellicane has given women a fantabulous gift! Part practical guide, part spiritual search engine, it contains everything a godly girlfriend needs to live fully, love freely, and finally take care of herself for a change. Get ready for 31 days of heavenly how-tos that will leave you inspired, invigorated, and in love with the Lord who made you beautiful—both inside and out."

—**Karen Ehman,** speaker for Proverbs 31 Ministries and Hearts
at Home Conferences; author of *A Life That Says Welcome* and
The Complete Guide to Getting and Staying Organized

"Arlene Pellicane's prescriptions for a younger you—heart, mind, and body—will inspire you toward a healthier lifestyle and a more youthful zest for life. Follow her practical tips and reflect on her daily encouragement for 31 days, and you will likely look and feel like a much younger woman!"

—**Danna Demetre, RN,** author of *Scale Down*
and *Change Your Habits, Change Your Life*

"In just 31 days Arlene Pellicane convinced me I can turn the clock back by taking just one step a day. Wow! Her positive words are so encouraging I may have to get out last month's calendar and relive it now that I am a younger me. Every woman with a busy life needs to get this book—and fast. After all, you don't want to waste the next 31 days aging before your time!"

—**Marcia Ramsland,** professional organizer and author of
Simplify Your Life; Simplify Your Time; and *Simplify Your Space.*

"Arlene Pellicane has written a comprehensive, holistic gift for all of us. No matter where you are in life, there is something in here to encourage you and help you to be all God dreams, desires and designed you to be. Thank you, Arlene!"

—**Sheila Schuller Coleman,** executive director of
Ministries and Missions, Crystal Cathedral

31 DAYS TO A YOUNGER YOU

Arlene Pellicane

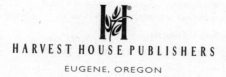

HARVEST HOUSE PUBLISHERS

EUGENE, OREGON

Cover design by Koechel Peterson and Associates, Inc., Minneapolis, Minnesota

Cover photo © iStockphoto/Thinkstock

Back cover author photo by Anthony Amorteguy

Readers are advised to consult with their physician or other medical practitioner before implementing the suggestions that follow. This book is not intended to take the place of sound professional medical advice or to treat specific maladies. Neither the author nor the publisher assumes any liability for possible adverse consequences as a result of the information contained herein.

31 Days to a Younger You
Copyright © 2010 by Arlene Pellicane
Published by Harvest House Publishers
Eugene, Oregon 97402
www.harvesthousepublishers.com

Library of Congress Cataloging-in-Publication Data
    Pellicane, Arlene, 1971-
    31 days to a younger you / Arlene Pellicane.
       p. cm.
    Includes bibliographical references.
    ISBN 978-0-7369-2903-5 (pbk.)
    1. Beauty, Personal—Religious aspects—Christianity. 2. Women—Health and hygiene.—Religious aspects—Christianity. 3. Rejuvenation—Religious aspects—Christianity. I. Title. II. Title: Thirty-one days to a younger you.
    RA778.P318 2010
    613'.04244—dc22

                                2010015981

Printed in the United States of America

11 12 13 14 15 16 17 18 19 / BP-SK / 10 9 8 7 6 5 4 3 2

To my husband, James
Thank you for believing in me.
I couldn't have done this without you.

To my children, Ethan, Noelle, and Lucy
Because I want to be young enough to play with your kids someday.

Contents

Foreword

I am writing this from Alaska, where I have been joined by many of my "Seasoned Sisters," ages 40 to almost 70. We have hiked a glacier and paddled the ocean bays with whales rising to greet us and eagles soaring overhead. We have met with God to read His words and hear His voice and His exciting calling—His adventure for our life's second half. The trip was planned as a celebration of the release of my book, *Woman of Confidence: Step into God's Adventure for Your Life*, and the end of my "jubilee" fiftieth birthday year. I am passionately in love with my husband, Bill, 31 years after the "I do." My three kids are grown, and the oldest has started a family of his own, so I am now affectionately called "Nana Go Go." And I feel *young*.

That's what Arlene Pellicane wants for you too. She wants you to create the best life possible. The wisdom in the pages of *31 Days to a Younger You* will help you feel young too.

I first met Arlene at a conference I was speaking at. She came to the "Hearts at Home" Mom's event with a dream on her heart, a dream to help encourage and equip women. She wants to help every reader squeeze the most she can out of what life offers and to live a life that pleases God. I remember being instantly impressed with Arlene. She is beautiful, smart, articulate, and passionate. Her years spent in television production rubbing shoulders with some of today's most influential leaders were well spent.

She was teachable then, gleaning wisdom from everyone she made contact with, but Arlene has deep wisdom of her own. She has created a loving, warm, passionate marriage with her husband. Her kids are healthy, happy, and well on the way to being leaders. Her friends look forward to time spent with her as we always come away a better person. Those under her ministry are living stronger and longer (and dare I say, thinner too).

Arlene models what she teaches. She is beautiful from the inside out, and she will show you how to do that too. She will also help you feel younger, dream younger, and have relationships that are reenergized, alive, and meaningful. You will leave this next 31 days healthier, and that just might make you wealthier, as you will have the energy and clarity to make the most of life's second half.

One might wonder what 31 days can do; after all, it's only a month. That's the secret. *31 Days to a Younger You* is packed with wisdom, activities, recommendations, examples, and easy to implement ideas that anyone can work into a busy life. Most of us live on the go, usually taking care of everyone else except ourselves. Arlene knows people today are fighting for a free moment to learn to enjoy life more and to live longer, and she has written this book so you can gain all you need in those snatches of time—in the moments waiting for the kids, the train, or for your ginkgo to kick in so you can find the car keys.

Arlene is a born cheerleader, and you will be motivated, encouraged, and excited to try all the helpful and realistic advice that will make your life better. Just think, in just one month you could feel like a new you!

On my desk and mirror where I put on my makeup each day are inspiring quotes, such as:

> "The glory of God is man fully alive."
> —St Irenaeus

> "It's never too late to be who you might have been."
> —George Eliot

> "I came that they may have life and have it abundantly."
> —Jesus (John 10:10)

Arlene Pellicane is a life coach, a cheerleader of change, and she can help you get to the abundant, full, exciting, meaningful, and rich plan for your life—one day at a time. Try it. Give it 31 days. I know you will see, as I did, that life can be better just 31 days from now—and every day after that too.

Pam Farrel
Relationship specialist, international speaker,
and author of over 30 books

Introduction

Turn Back the Clock

I t was a beautiful summer day on the beach. The beachfront teemed with kids building sand castles, bikini-clad teens, parasailers, and even a few dolphins. But what stood out to me the most were two middle-aged women who ran with all their might into the Atlantic, splashing and laughing as though they were 14 again. They were probably in their forties, but they didn't look it. They were moving too fast, laughing too hard, and looking too silly to be women in midlife.

Or were they? Who says midlife has to be predictable, inactive, or boring? Your forties and beyond are a time to celebrate being comfortable in your own skin (even if it's more wrinkly than it used to be). It's time to step out into new adventures, embrace change, treasure your family, look and feel better than ever.

Women over the age of 40 are 78 million strong in the United States,[1] but some are harder than others to spot. Celebrities such as Julia Roberts, Jennifer Aniston, and Halle Berry aren't the only ones looking ten years younger. Ordinary women are doing it too.

Well, you may think, *those women have good genes. And personal trainers. And lots of money.* Although that may be true, there are several things *any* woman can do to look and feel younger without spending any money. In the next 31 days, how would you like to:

- Be thinner and more attractive

- Wake up with excitement for life

- Have more energy to do what you want

- Update your wardrobe without looking as if you're trying too hard

- Improve your relationship with your spouse, children, family, and friends

- Master daily habits that improve the quantity and quality of your days

All of this is possible if you'll make the commitment to take an honest look in the mirror, both at your body and soul, and allow God to touch your life from the inside out.

If God Looks at the Heart, Why Do the Other Parts Matter?

If God cares only about the inner life, you may wonder why bother with makeup, haircuts, or weight-loss programs? In fact, why can't you stay in pajamas all day if you want? One answer is found in a core value my husband read to me, "Excellence as the minimum standard." As a beloved child of God, you don't want to go through life with the opposite motto, "Doing the minimum is good enough."

So why not dedicate your heart to God as the minimum, but then strive for excellence in other areas of your life as well? Give God everything, which includes your heart, mind, *and* body. I've met some people who believe if you care about your appearance, you're vain and misdirected since God looks at the inside, not the outside, of a person. That could be true if you care *too much* about your appearance, but otherwise it can easily serve as a cop-out for laziness. Outward beauty and godliness aren't mutually exclusive qualities. Think both/and, not either/or. It's possible for you to be attractive *and* holy at the same time. No question that the higher priority should be placed on your inner life, but there's virtue in taking care of your physical being as well. Your family will certainly appreciate your efforts to look your best—especially your husband if you're married.

My friend Jane became a card-carrying member of Medicare this year, although she looks a decade younger. She's a classy lady with a quick step and ready smile. Whenever I see her, she's impeccably dressed and her makeup is perfect. When I asked about her motivation for putting her best foot forward, Jane said, "I am a royal princess in God's kingdom. He has given me this temple (my body), and I must treat it well. If He really is my king and I am His daughter, I should look a certain way. An ambassador should bring honor to the one he or she represents."[2]

Beauty does come from the inside out—but people see your outsides first. When you do all you can to look your best, you honor your King and Creator, and that's why all the other parts really do matter.

How the Nursing Home Changed My Life

When I was in my late twenties, I was single without a prospect in sight. I longed to be married and regularly asked God to send along Mr. Wonderful. My prayers were answered in an unusual place: smack dab in the middle of a nursing home. While in graduate school, I enjoyed participating in an outreach to the local nursing home on Friday nights. We would sing in the activity center, share a Bible story, and then visit individuals in their rooms. One Friday, a young man named James shared the Bible story. The seniors may not have been hanging on his every word, but I certainly was.

I'm happy to say James and I are married today. We laugh that we started in a nursing home, and we may end up there one day too. But between those two experiences, there's a whole lot of living to do. We have three children under the age of six, so my kids are three major motivations for me to look and feel younger. I want to be able to hike together through the Grand Canyon when they're young adults, or dance at their weddings someday. That's why I've interviewed women in their fifties, sixties—and even a 100-year-old who still drives and lives on her own—to find out their secrets for longevity. In the coming chapters, you'll get great advice from former Women of Faith speaker Thelma Wells, organizing pro Marcia Ramsland, bestselling author Pam Farrel, life coach Danna Demetre, and many more extraordinary women.

I'd like you to take a moment right now to consider your motivation for looking and feeling younger. Do you have it? Whether you want to turn your husband's head, gain more confidence, live with less pain, try for that promotion at work, or look fantastic for your upcoming high-school reunion, this book can help you get there.

Getting the Most Out of This Book

I must warn you that sleeping with this book under your pillow will do nothing for your crow's-feet, and reading a chapter about exercise won't make you lose an inch of belly fat. The transformation begins to happen when you *do something* about what you're reading. This book is divided into three sections because these facets of your life are important components to looking and feeling younger:

Days 1–9: Your Personal Rx for the Heart

Days 10–16: Your Personal Rx for the Mind

Days 17–31: Your Personal Rx for the Body

Beauty is about much more than Botox and diets, but it's not confined to the invisible places of the heart either. This book has been written with the busy woman in mind so you'll be able to finish each daily reading and reflection in five to ten minutes. You may choose to read it in 31 consecutive days, or you may want to take a break on the weekends, and finish the book in six weeks. This is your personal guide, so do whatever works for you.

The only thing I ask is that you don't skip the personal prescription (*Rx*) for change at the end of each chapter.

The R stands for Rejuvenation. Rejuvenation means to make young again, to restore to youthful vigor and appearance. In this daily feature, we'll consider what would rejuvenate you in a particular area of life.

The X stands for eXpression. This section is about how you're going to take the information in each chapter and use it in your life. Completing each daily action step is one of the most important components to your success.

My father is a family physician, so whenever I got sick growing up, I could always count on him to write me a prescription for what I needed. Of course that little piece of paper didn't do anything for my cold. I had to take the medicine. In the same way, just reading the action steps at the end of each chapter won't cure any of what ails you. To look and feel younger, do yourself a favor. Read this book with a pencil or pen in hand, and be ready for action. Don't despise small beginnings; it's the small, incremental changes that last.

Get Ready for Your Makeover

One of my favorite motivational speakers, Zig Ziglar, says that many people are poor learners because they focus on acquiring more knowledge instead of applying what they already know.[3] Did you catch that? There's a life-changing difference between *knowing what to do* and *actually doing it*.

The ball is in your court. Be an optimist for the next 31 days and take action on what you read. If you do, you will look and feel younger, guaranteed. Some results will be immediate, others will take a few months, and still others may be fully enjoyed only in eternity.

- Short-term change = You get a new flattering haircut, outfit, or pair of hip glasses.

- Long-term change = You lose 20 pounds through healthier eating and exercise.

- Eternal change = You find new joy in the Lord and learn to let go of a critical spirit.

So are you ready for your 31-day journey? It's time to turn back the clock and move forward as a younger, happier you.

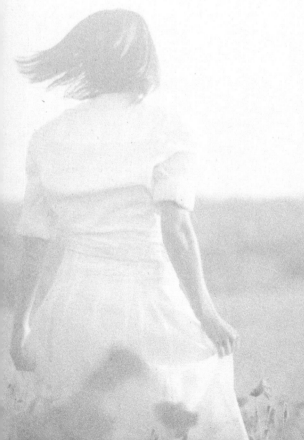

Your Personal Rx for the Heart

Above all else, guard your heart,
for it is the wellspring of life.

PROVERBS 4:23

Back to First Grade

I f you could go back in time, would you?

Most of us would pass because we remember the pain of puberty, high-school breakups, and dreadful first jobs. But what about those carefree kindergarten days when every morning brought a new chance to play?

My parents were born and raised in Indonesia, and they immigrated to New York before I was born. Shoveling snow was getting to my father, so when I was six, my family moved from New York to California. I tested out of first grade and began my new school as a second grader. Most people never knew I was younger than the other kids because I was tall.

Now that I have children, I wonder if there's anything I missed by skipping first grade. First graders learn about addition and subtraction of whole numbers. They become masters of the alphabet, learning all the sounds and reading easy books. They are learning basic fundamentals and having lots of fun in the process.

Is it possible to learn the fundamentals of anything and have fun in the process? Sure, just look at little kids. Their eyes sparkle when shown a new object. They giggle with delight over simple stories. The word *fundamental* actually begins with *fun*. Have you ever looked at that word in that way? One definition of fundamental is "relating to the foundation or base, forming or serving as an essential component of a system or structure, or something that is an essential or necessary part of a system or object."[1] As you were reading that definition, you probably weren't thinking, *Wow, that sounds exciting!*

Practicing fundamentals may seem tedious, boring, and laborious. But therein lies one secret to looking and feeling younger: injecting *fun* into the *fun*damentals.

Can We Read the Bible, Please?

My kindergartener, Ethan, loves to read his Bible. He comes into my room in the morning asking, "Mommy, can you read me a story from the Bible?" His Bible is written as a children's storybook with colorful illustrations and animated characters. Whether the story is "David and Goliath" or "Jesus Feeds Thousands," Ethan's attention is sharply fixed on each page. After one story has ended, he wants another, then another.

I sometimes wish I had this same kind of hunger and enthusiasm when I approach my Bible. I'd like to read it with fresh eyes like my son's. Instead of knowing how things turn out, what if I read a story about Jesus and wondered, *What's going to happen? Is Jesus really going to walk on water? How did He do that?*

If you're not careful, Bible study can become a chore, something to check off a "to-do" list and nothing more. Anyone can become numb to the miraculous stories and truths found in God's Word. After sharing a parable in Mark 7, Jesus says to His closest followers, "Are you so dull?" (Mark 7:18). Even the disciples who walked with Jesus experienced times of spiritual blindness.

Reading the Bible is a fundamental component to living your best life, yet so many people have forgotten the fun—the life—that's found in studying God's Word. So how do you put the fun back into the fundamentals of Bible study?

Pray first. Before you begin reading, take a moment to ask God to help you comprehend and apply what you read, that "the eyes of your heart may be enlightened in order that you may know the hope to which he has called you, the riches of his glorious inheritance in the saints, and his incomparably great power for us who believe" (Ephesians 1:18-19).

Personalize it. When you read an Old Testament story, put yourself in the picture. What if you instead of Daniel were thrown inside the lion's den? How would you feel when the morning came and you were still alive? You can also insert your name into a passage: "[Mary] be kind and compassionate to one another, forgiving each other, just as in Christ God forgave you" (Ephesians 4:32).

Put it into practice. If you love to play basketball, it's enjoyable to watch a game on television but not nearly as fun as suiting up and playing yourself. Likewise, you can sit on the sidelines, observing the truths found in the Bible. But until you put what you read into practice, you're not fully realizing the positive power of God's Word in your life. Take a passage of Scripture and ask God how to apply it to your life.

Here's a beauty tip that illustrates what reading the Bible will do for you. To give your makeup a firm base, splash your face with cold water before applying makeup. This helps shrink pores temporarily and helps makeup glide on seamlessly.

When you read your Bible, it's like splashing cold, refreshing water on your face. It cleanses your life of imperfections. It shrinks not your pores but your problems. It gives you fresh energy for the day. When you apply makeup, it helps your outward appearance. But applying God's Word dramatically improves your inward appearance where true beauty begins.

I may be too old to sit in a first-grade classroom, but I'm young enough at heart to have fun doing the fundamentals, and so are you.

Thought for Rejuvenation

Think back to a time when Bible study was especially meaningful to you. Maybe you were studying a particular book, using a study guide, or looking for answers during a difficult time of life. What were you doing that worked well?

Act of eXpression

Do something today to make your Bible study come alive. Here are a few ideas:

- Read the Bible with a notepad. Write your thoughts about a few passages and how they apply to your life.

- Pray a few Scriptures out loud, inserting your name when appropriate.

- Listen to an audio Bible on CD or your computer.

- Take your Bible to a quiet place outside and read in a different environment than usual.

The Joy Factor

Think of a woman who looks younger than she really is. What does she look like? Is she cheerful and optimistic or sullen and serious? Most likely the woman you pictured is smiling broadly, exuding joy wherever she goes. When she walks into a room, people can't help but notice her 1000-watt smile and natural charisma.

When you boil it down, looking young is about looking healthy and *happy*. But wait a minute. Isn't happiness an emotion you feel only when things go your way? Isn't a happy life something out of your control, reserved only for the lucky ones who get the best breaks?

In his book, *Happiness Is a Serious Problem*, author and radio talk-show host Dennis Prager writes:

> The notion that happiness must be constantly worked at comes as news, disconcerting news, to many people. They assume that happiness is a feeling and that this feeling comes as a result of good things that happen to them. We therefore have little control over how happy we are, the thinking goes, because we can control neither how we feel nor what happens to us. This book is predicated on the opposite premise: Happiness is largely, though certainly not entirely, determined by us, through hard work (most particularly by controlling our nature) and through attaining wisdom (developing attitudes that enable us not to despair).[2]

The Bible says it this way in Habakkuk 3:18, "I will be joyful in God my Savior." Living with joy and happiness is a choice, an act of one's will rather than a haphazard emotion.

Consider my two-year-old daughter, Noelle. Like all toddlers, she over-reacts—if she is served milk in the green cup instead of the pink cup, she might go ballistic. But my husband, James, has taught her that whenever she throws a fit, she doesn't get what she wants. Instead, she's instructed to stop crying, ask nicely for what she wants with no whining, and even smile. James says, "Let me see your happy face," and she shrivels up her face in the fakest smile you can imagine. But at least she's trying. If a two-year-old can learn to act happy, even when she doesn't feel like it, certainly you can too.

Happiness is not only an active choice of the will; it's a commandment for the Christian. We're instructed to "be joyful always" (1 Thessalonians 5:16). The Amplified Version says it this way, "Be happy [in your faith] and rejoice and be glad-hearted continually (always)," and the Message says, "Be cheerful no matter what...this is the way God wants you who belong to Christ Jesus to live" (vv. 16,18).

Living Sunny-Side Up

I have an edge when it comes to living cheerfully because I was raised by the happiest person I know, my mother. Mom doesn't walk, she bounces. You hear her laughing and talking happily long before you see her. Growing up, my friends would always ask me, "Is your mom *always* this happy?" to which I would reply without hesitation, "Yes."

She turned 60 this year, and once in a while people will still ask if we're sisters. The source of my mother's youth isn't in her skin (she has age spots) or figure (she's not a size six). It's the joy factor. Her vitality radiates from her face—those bright eyes and that unstoppable smile.

I think my mom was born sunny-side up, but she's also made choices in life that every woman can make to live happily ever after.

- Rejoice in the Lord and keep your focus on Him, not your circumstances.

- Believe the best about everyone.

- Don't hold onto grudges.

- Champion the underdog.

- Look for ways to minister to others.

- Laugh often.

Ironman Strength

This year, my family had the opportunity to watch part of an Ironman 70.3 triathlon. Ironman 70.3 races include a 1.2-mile swim, a 56-mile bike ride, and a 13.1-mile run. We saw numerous 40- and 50-somethings cross the finish line, and even a 69-year-old, but we were most inspired by the man using a racing wheelchair. He had no legs and was powering through those hot, rigorous miles using his upper body alone. As we cheered wildly for him, he looked up and stuck out his tongue as if to say, "Phew, this is tough." But the twinkle in his eye revealed his joy. From joy comes great strength.

How's your strength level today? You may or may not be ready to train for a triathlon, but do you live with a twinkle in your eye like that inspiring athlete in the wheelchair? The journey to looking younger begins within. Remember the beautiful words of hope found in Nehemiah 8:10, "Do not grieve, for the joy of the LORD is your strength."

Thought for Rejuvenation

Read this Scripture aloud:

> The LORD appeared to us in the past, saying:
>   "I have loved you with an everlasting love;
>   I have drawn you with loving-kindness.
>   I will build you up again
>   and you will be rebuilt, O Virgin Israel.
>   Again you will take up your tambourines
>   and go out to dance with the joyful."
>   (Jeremiah 31:3-4)

Write down one way God has loved you and shown you loving-kindness this week.

Act of eXpression

What's one thing you can do today to exude more joy in your life?

MY SEVEN FAVORITE FOODS TO BOOST YOUR MOOD

Oatmeal is packed with soluble fiber to lower blood sugar levels and reduce irritability.

Whole-Grain Bread contains a wide variety of the amino acids needed to keep your mood upbeat.

Salmon has omega-3 fatty acids that are used by the brain to produce neurotransmitters to stave off depression and repair brain cells needed to boost your mood.

Chicken has a high level of tyrosine, an amino acid that helps elevate levels of norepinephrine and dopamine. These chemicals are involved in the reaction time of your body, the motivation you feel, and possibly depression.

Leafy Greens are an excellent source of folic acid, a lack of which has been linked to depressed mood.

Milk is a great feel-good drink because calcium can help reduce your levels of stress and anxiety, and it contains tryptophan that helps your body produce serotonin, which elevates mood.

Bananas also contain tryptophan, plus they're packed with potassium and vitamin B6 to regulate blood sugar and stabilize mood.

You're Soaking in It

Do you remember the Palmolive commercials with Madge the manicurist? Madge was famous for soaking her customers' fingernails in Palmolive dishwashing liquid during their chatty visits at the local beauty parlor. The phrases, "You're soaking in it" and "Palmolive soften hands while you do the dishes," are a few of the most recognized television commercial quotes of all time.

Instead of soaking in dishwashing soap to soften your hands, wouldn't it be nice to find a way to soak in God's Word to soften your heart? Could it be as simple as sitting quietly, not with your manicurist but with the Lord?

After I graduated from college, I got a job and rented a room from one of my favorite college professors. One thing I remember is the picture of her sitting in the same chair every morning with her Bible open. Her time with the Lord was consistent, precious to her, and an incredible example to me of resting in God's presence. She never seemed hurried or anxious; her life was rooted and grounded in Christ every morning. Her home was a sanctuary of peace and praise.

Today, Satan does some of his best work by keeping Christians busy. Busyness in itself is not a sin, but running around from morning till night, finally flopping on our beds, too pooped to pray must surely displease God. The idea of waiting quietly—even for five minutes—to hear His voice seems strangely foreign in our frenetic world.

Why Bother to Meditate?

Meditation has been wrongly categorized by many as an activity reserved for super Christians or New Age enthusiasts. But Christian meditation is commanded in Scripture for every believer. The psalmist says of the person who is blessed, "But his delight is in the law of the LORD, and on his law he *meditates* day and night" (Psalm 1:2). Joshua 1:8 says it this way: "Do not let this Book of the Law depart from your mouth; *meditate* on it day and night, so that you may be careful to do everything written in it. Then you will be prosperous and successful." These Scriptures weren't written for the extra-spiritual Christian; they were written for *every* Christian. After all, don't you want to be prosperous and successful?

Meditation 101

The word *meditation* means to muse, ponder, rehearse in one's mind, or contemplate. So how does one ponder the truth found in God's Word?

- Read the Bible slowly, not rushing through the verses.

- Put yourself in the Scripture when possible. Be there. Feel the heat of the sun. Hear the crowd shouting.

- Pick one verse (or phrase) that stands out in your mind.

- Think about this verse throughout your day. Write it on an index card and put it somewhere you will see it. Rehearse the verse in your mind while you're waiting or driving.

- Can you draw a picture that reminds you of the verse?

- Tell someone about the verse you're meditating on. Ask for that person's insights.

- Have you ever experienced something that illustrates the verse?

- Pray about the verse.

- Think about the verse before you go to bed and when you wake up in the morning.

I like how Rick Warren describes meditation: "Meditation is *focused* thinking. It takes serious effort. You select a verse and reflect on it over and over in your mind...if you know how to worry, you already know how to meditate...No other habit can do more to transform your life and make you more like Jesus than daily reflection on Scripture."[3]

As you allow your heart and mind to soak in God's Word, you'll see a noticeable difference in your life. You'll begin to act more like Christ. This focus on obedience is what most clearly distinguishes Christian meditation from its Eastern and secular counterparts. Richard Foster writes that "Christian meditation, very simply, is the ability to hear God's voice and obey his word. It involves no hidden mysteries, no secret mantras, no mental gymnastics, no esoteric flights into the cosmic consciousness."[4]

Notice these important differences between Christian meditation and Eastern or secular meditation:

Christian Meditation	Eastern Meditation
Seeks to be filled with God's Spirit	Seeks to empty one's self
Focuses on God	Focuses on self
Rehearses Scriptures	Rehearses mantras
Results in changed behavior	Results in higher self-consciousness

Comfort Food

Women in midlife often struggle with relationships. You find out your college-age son is sexually active. Your aging parents need your care. Your husband is going through his own midlife crisis. And the women's committee at church is asking you to head up a major ministry. When life gets tough, the tough often head to the refrigerator. What if instead of turning to physical food for comfort, you turned to the spiritual food found in the Bible?

Try chewing on these verses instead of diving into your favorite comfort food:

When your children are rebelling:

Teach [my child], O LORD, to follow your decrees;
    then [he/she] will keep them to the end.
Give [my child] understanding to keep your law
    and obey it with all [his/her] heart.
Direct [my child] in the path of your commands,
    for there [he/she will] find delight.

Turn [my child] toward your statutes
and not toward selfish gain.
(Psalm 119:33-36)

When your husband is unresponsive:

Wives, in the same way be submissive to your husbands so that, if any of them do not believe the word, they may be won over without words by the behavior of their wives, when they see the purity and reverence of your lives (1 Peter 3:1-2).

When your parents are aging:

If a widow has children or grandchildren, these should learn first of all to put their religion into practice by caring for their own family and so repaying their parents and grandparents, for this is pleasing to God (1 Timothy 5:4).

When your work is monotonous:

Whatever you do, work at it with all your heart, as working for the Lord, not for men, since you know that you will receive an inheritance from the Lord as a reward. It is the Lord Christ you are serving (Colossians 3:23-24).

When your heart is heavy:

Cast all your anxiety on him because he cares for you (1 Peter 5:7).

Better Than Palmolive

Try this simple exercise called "palms down, palms up" from *The Celebration of Discipline* by Richard Foster. Begin with your palms down, symbolizing your desire to turn over your concerns to God. You may pray something like, "Lord, I give you my anxiety about my finances." Release that burden to the Lord and wait in surrender to Him. Then turn your palms up slowly as a symbol of your desire to receive from the Lord. You might pray, "Lord, I would like to receive your divine blessings on my finances. Please provide enough for everything we need this month." Spend the remaining moments in silence, allowing the Lord to comfort you and commune with you.[5]

Soaking in Palmolive may help you get softer skin, but doing exercises such as "palms down, palms up" will help soften your heart to hear God speaking to you. Meditating on God's Word will strengthen your soul, life, and relationships—and you don't have to go to a beauty salon to get started.

BEAUTY TIP

Let your moisturizer soak in. Give your facial lotion time to completely absorb, about three minutes, before applying makeup. This will help foundation, blush, and shadow last all day.

Thought for Rejuvenation

Do you meditate on God's Word? What are some ways you can soak regularly in the Scriptures?

Act of eXpression

Take one of the verses from today's reading and meditate on it. Use one or more of the ideas found earlier in this chapter under Meditation 101.

Day 4

Heart-Healthy Choices

The familiar phrase "Bless your heart" has taken on a whole new meaning for Pamela Christian. One morning at age 47, Pamela went to play tennis with three other ladies. She arrived with a feeling of indigestion and chalked it up to the cantaloupe she'd been eating. During the warm-up, she was hitting the ball in every direction except where it was supposed to go. Embarrassed and unusually short of breath, she decided to rest and then go home. Before she could get to her car, she threw up and couldn't muster the strength to walk. Her breathing was shallow, and as she lay on the sidewalk, her tennis partners called 911.

When the paramedics arrived, they immediately administered life-saving procedures because Pamela was experiencing sudden cardiac arrest. Her heart had abruptly stopped. The paramedics shocked her with a defibrillator and put an oxygen mask on her face, and her heart began beating again.

At the hospital, the doctors could not figure out why Pamela suffered cardiac arrest. Weight wasn't a problem; she didn't smoke or have a history of heart disease in her family. There wasn't an electrical problem or an obstruction in the arteries around her heart. After surviving her dramatic and unexpected cardiac arrest (95 percent of those who suffer sudden cardiac arrest don't survive), Pamela founded a ministry called "Bless Your Heart" (www.blessyourheartcampaign.com) to increase awareness among women about heart disease. With great passion, she urges women to examine their lifestyle and make the necessary changes to reduce their risk.[6]

How Does Your Heart Rate?

Here are a few questions to quickly assess your heart health:

- Do you eat a well-balanced, healthy diet?

- Do you exercise regularly?

- Do you smoke or use recreational drugs?

- Are your blood pressure, weight, and diabetes (if applicable) under control?

- Do you manage depression effectively?

Feel convicted in any of these areas? Here are two simple things you can do today to radically improve your heart health.

Go Mediterranean: Eat olive oil, leafy greens, whole grains, nuts, fruit, fish, tomatoes, salmon, and other foods with omega-3s.

Go Active: Exercise at least 10 minutes a day and aim for 30 minutes daily.

According to the American Heart Association, a complete physical fitness program should include activities that promote *endurance*, *strength*, and *flexibility*.[7] To build endurance, do aerobic activities such as brisk walking, running, cycling, or swimming. To build strength, try weight lifting. You can lift weights at the gym or you can buy a set of 5-, 10-, and 15-pound dumbbells to use at home. To improve flexibility, do stretching and movements that put each part of the body through its full range of motion.

What form of exercise has the lowest dropout rate? If you guessed walking, you're right. Walking is free, easy, and convenient. No special equipment is necessary, though it's advisable to invest in a good pair of walking shoes. Whether you're 45 or 65, you can walk year-round, though in some climates you may want to walk indoors, perhaps at an indoor shopping mall, during winter months. Walking is low impact so your risk of injury to bones and joints is minimal.

Your overall fitness goal is a body mass index (BMI) of 18.5–24.9. BMI is a measure of body fat based on height and weight. Just search for "BMI calculator" on the Internet and input your height and weight to discover your personal BMI.

Another way to easily assess your cardiovascular health is by taking your resting heart rate. Take your pulse at the thumb side of your wrist after sitting calmly for at least five minutes or when you wake up in the morning. Count the beats for ten seconds, then multiply that number by six to determine how many beats per minute. Your resting pulse should be no higher than eighty beats per minute. If your resting pulse is high, your heart needs some extra TLC. Talk to your doctor about improving your diet and adding cardiovascular exercise. Because the heart is a muscle, exercise such as running or cycling will make it stronger.

Does Your Heart Beat for God?

To look and feel younger, not only should your heart be strong physically, it must be strong spiritually. Are you smitten with Jesus Christ? Are you in love with your Savior? I remember falling in love with my husband, James. Whenever he came into the room, my heart started beating wildly and butterflies swirled in my stomach. Throughout our courtship and up to today, my heart was and is completely his.

Does this describe your relationship with Jesus Christ? Do you love Him tenderly, with passion and devotion? Deuteronomy 6:5 tells us to "Love the LORD your God with all your heart and with all your soul and with all your strength."

The Hot Heart

Elizabeth George in her book, *A Woman After God's Own Heart,* writes, "Our heart for God should be like a boiling pot. Our heart should be characterized by God-given and intense emotion and passion for our Lord. After all, when a teakettle is boiling on your stove, you know it!"[8]

If you need some help rekindling the flame between you and God, why not write Him a love letter? Write out the characteristics you appreciate about God, thank Him for specific blessings, and pour out your concerns to Him. Listen to worship music that both touches your heart and communicates what you want to say to God. Think back to a time when you felt very close to Christ. What was happening in your life? How was your heart hotter toward God then? Pray and ask God to help you return to that first love.

The Trusting Heart

When my son Ethan was three years old, he was very afraid of going into a swimming pool. The moment his little toe touched the water, he was already screaming, "*Out! Out!* I want *out!*" But in time—and with a lot of coaxing—he could handle being in the shallow end of the pool (clinging to his daddy, of course).

One day, James instructed Ethan to stand at the edge of the pool and jump into his arms. Ethan stood there, his feet solidly cemented to the ground. He wasn't going anywhere. "Look into my eyes and trust me," his daddy said. "I won't let you fall." With great faith and his eyes half closed, my little boy flung himself into his father's arms. There were a few tears, but he survived. Every time he jumped, it got easier.

This picture reminds me of what it's like to trust God. Sometimes it feels like jumping into the great unknown, hoping there will be a safety net. Rest assured; your heavenly Father will always catch you, and the more you jump, the easier it will get.

The Obedient Heart

Have you ever had a two-year-old child or grandchild stare you in the face, stand toe-to-toe with you, and declare with unbridled boldness, "*No!*" Usually the "No!" is accompanied with excessive crying, whining, screaming, and maybe a temper tantrum. When you think of it, a disobedient child is terribly unhappy.

Do you want a happy heart, one that feels youthful and light? Then learn to obey God in the big and small matters of life. In Acts 13:22, David was described as a man after God's own heart: "I have found David son of Jesse a man after my own heart; *he will do everything I want him to do.*" David's heart was praised because of his obedience.

I hope you can say with the psalmist,

> Your statutes are my heritage forever;
>   they are the joy of my heart.
> My heart is set on keeping your decrees
>   to the very end.
>   (Psalm 119:111-112)

When your heart is *hot* for God, *trusts* Him completely, and is *obedient*, you will make choices that will bless your heart both today and in eternity.

Thought for Rejuvination

How would you describe the state of your heart? Are you critical, fearful, indifferent, cynical, childlike, excited, peaceful, happy?

My heart is:

A Prayer for Today: Lord, I give You my heart. Help me to have the discipline to take care of my physical heart with exercise and healthy eating. Your Word says to guard my heart for out of it come the springs of life (Proverbs 4:23). Guard my heart from destructive habits. Cleanse my heart from sin and make me aware of any sin that's keeping me from You. I want my heart to burn brightly for You. Help me to trust and obey You each day. Others may look at my outward appearance, but I know You look at the heart (1 Samuel 16:7). So may my heart be pleasing before You.

Act of eXpression

To get some idea of your physical heart health, you can take a free online risk assessment at the website for the American Heart Association (www.americanheart.org). But always check with your doctor for a more thorough assessment.

What is one thing you can do today to improve your heart health **spiritually?**

The Warmth of Community

Have you ever attended a women's retreat and felt left out? For Tami, the thought of spending the weekend with 70 other women was not her idea of a good time. She'd much rather go on a fishing trip with a bunch of guys than spend the weekend with emotional women talking about menopause, the latest sale at Nordstrom, and other useless small talk. But as newcomers to the church, her husband urged her to go and make some friends. Reluctantly she agreed.

The day of the retreat, she stood at the registration table with that sinking feeling she had made a mistake. She was assigned a room with three other women she didn't know. She didn't recognize any faces around her. Tami quickly retreated into her car, called her husband, and started to cry. She wanted to go home, but her husband encouraged her to stay. She walked back into the meeting room and quietly found a seat.

Fast forward to the end of the retreat. I was the speaker that weekend, and when the women were asked what God had done in their lives, Tami was among the first to speak up. She had tears in her eyes again, but this time they were tears of joy. She said,

> I didn't want to come here. I used to be in ministry, but then I fell and felt like God could not use me anymore. This weekend, God has shown me I can still minister to others. A woman prayed for me and quoted a verse in Jeremiah, the exact verse that was prayed over me when I was called into ministry. My three roommates made me feel so welcome. God's Word says "He sets the

solitary in families" (Psalm 68:6 NKJV) and that's exactly what He did for me at this retreat. I feel part of a family.[9]

Today Tami is active in her church community, singing in the choir, and sharing her contagious laughter with everyone around her. Being part of a happy and healthy church community has made all the difference in the world.

Be a Seasoned Sister

Are you experiencing the warmth of community in your church? In a Bible study or small group? In a knitting or book club? At your workplace? Whether you play bridge or Bunco with friends, or the piano in a worship band, you need a place to make meaningful connections with others to feel younger and more alive.

My mentor, Pam Farrel, understands this so well she founded an organization called Seasoned Sisters. Seasoned Sisters encourages women to meet in personal support groups to help them live a fantastic life after 40. The name is "seasoned" because these women are old enough to know what they want out of life and wise enough to know what to do with those dreams. "Sisters" because when women stand shoulder-to-shoulder, they are stronger—as when a builder hammers a wall stud or floor joist to an existing stud or joist to strengthen it (called *sistering*).

Here's how one Seasoned Sister, Vickie, describes the warmth of community she's experienced:

> My closest friends, women that I trust and admire the most, have been those I met or got to know better through Seasoned Sisters. It is a safe place—one where I feel accepted and encouraged to grow, both in my faith and my personal life. Life was not meant to be experienced alone. The hard times are much less difficult when we have close friends beside us. This stage of life is full of changes and challenges such as empty nest, health issues, and retirement. Seasoned Sisters provides a place for Christian women to laugh, share, and be encouraged.[10]

Pick Your Friends Wisely

You'll pick up attitudes and habits (both good and bad) from your closest friends, so choose wisely. If you surround yourself with women who constantly complain about their aches, pains, and problems, that's not going to help you feel younger. When interviewed on the *Today* show, Dan Buettner, author of *The Blue Zones: Lessons for Living Longer from the People Who've Lived the Longest*, said,

> If your three best friends are obese, there's a 50 percent chance or better that you'll be overweight and you'll live less. So if you think about who you hang out with, hang out with people whose idea of physical activity is recreation...It will naturally influence you over the long run, a much more powerful longevity supplement than any pill you can take.[11]

Are you choosing the kind of friends who will challenge you to be physically fit, mentally active, and spiritually engaged?

Is Facebook for Me?

One way to find a community of like-minded friends is through social networking on the Internet. Women older than 55 make up the fastest growing age group on the popular social networking website Facebook. About 1.5 million female users over 55 are on the site, roughly a 550 percent increase from just six months prior.[12] Think of Facebook as an electronic directory of names, photo album, and living room rolled into one. It's easy to use and free to sign up. All you need is an email address to begin.

Mothers and grandmothers are logging on to see what their children and grandchildren are up to. Your grandson may not be very talkative when you call him, but you can find out a lot about his interests by reading his Facebook page. You can have meaningful chitchat with your teenage daughter or granddaughter simply by typing in comments and questions.

Besides your family, you can get in contact with high school class-mates and former coworkers by entering their names in a people search or entering your school and date of graduation. I have found favorite college professors, kids I grew up with in upstate New York, and coworkers from earlier days.

An online community can help you keep in touch with friends and loved ones and introduce you to new people with similar interests and values. If you're not sure how to do all this on the computer, have no fear. You can have some bonding time with your son, daughter, grandchild, niece, or nephew as they teach you how to use it.

Designed for Community

As convenient as the computer is (you can read the latest scoop on your friends and family without even getting out of your pajamas), nothing can replace meeting others face-to-face. The Bible encourages us in Hebrews 10:24-25, "Let us consider how we may spur one another on toward love and good deeds. Let us not give up meeting together, as some are in the habit of doing, but let us encourage one another—and all the more as you see the Day approaching."

Experiencing the warmth of community isn't just a happy ideal; it's a biblical principle for life. Disillusioned by the local church, many believers have turned inward, choosing to worship God from home rather than in a traditional congregation. But there's a downside to this isolationism. We were designed to live most effectively in community.

My mom always taught me to look for someone who needed a friend whenever I went to church. If I sought to be a friend first to others, I would never be lonely myself. Whenever I feel anxiety before walking into a room of strangers, I remember my mother's advice. When you take the first step to be friendly to others, you'll find the caring community you crave—and you'll never attend a women's retreat and feel left out!

BEAUTY TIP:

To achieve a natural glow on your face, rub your palms together for a minute, then press them gently across your face after applying foundation. The warmth of your hands helps soften the foundation, making it look like your natural skin instead of an obvious layer of makeup.

Thought for Rejuvenation

What communities do you belong in (church, Sunday school class, small groups, clubs, professional associations, hobby groups)?

Do you feel a regular and meaningful connection with a group of women?

Act of eXpression

Make a commitment to be active in a community:

- Join a small group at church
- Start a women's Bible study in your home
- Join or begin a Seasoned Sisters group (www.seasonedsisters.com)
- Start your Facebook page (www.facebook.com)
- Attend a professional networking group

What will you do in the next 31 days to be active in a community?

Grace in a Bottle

When you think of a timeless beauty, perhaps Grace Kelly comes to mind. The accomplished and beautiful actress has been upheld as a standard for poise, elegance, and style. In 1956, she married Prince Rainier Grimaldi III of Monaco to become Princess Grace of Monaco. Royalty suited her well.

I know another beautiful Grace who is not as famous as Princess Grace, but she is royalty as well—a child of the King.

When I was working as a features producer for the *700 Club*, one of my first interviews was with a courageous double amputee named Gracie Rosenberger. Believe it or not, we went rock climbing together at an indoor gym. I figured if a double amputee could scale up a wall, I should be able to follow. Despite her physical obstacles, Gracie kept living to the fullest—rock climbing, skiing, and playing basketball with her husband and two boys.

In her wildest dreams, Gracie never pictured her life without legs. As a college music major in 1983, she had her sights set on Nashville and singing stardom. But that all changed one night when she fell asleep at the wheel. Her car slammed into a concrete abutment, flipped, and rolled into a gully. Her car burst into flames. Her legs were crushed and pushed over her shoulders.

"I remember thinking, I can't move my body and I can't get out of here," Gracie says. "I was going to die unless the Lord intervened."

She was rescued by some truckers who saw the accident. When she arrived at the hospital, she had lost so much blood that her blood pressure was 40 over 20. Three weeks later, she woke up in a hospital bed with searing pain and a broken body and soul.

As of this writing, Gracie's had 72 operations, including the amputation of her right leg in 1991 and the left in 1995. There hasn't been one day since the accident when Gracie hasn't experienced physical pain. But she found the key to living with grace in Paul's words in 2 Corinthians 12:9, "'My grace is sufficient for you, for my power is made perfect in weakness.' Therefore I will boast all the more gladly about my weaknesses, so that Christ's power may rest on me." Gracie sees her weakness as an avenue for God's grace to flood her life.[13]

With her husband, Peter, and sons, Parker and Grayson, Gracie has traveled to Ghana, West Africa, to provide prosthetic limbs for amputees. Gracie's organization, Standing with Hope, offers the supplies and training necessary to build quality prosthetics, a gift that changes someone's life forever. Gracie recalls,

> While recovering from having my remaining leg amputated, I watched a documentary showing the plight of amputees in developing countries and instantly knew my calling. Lying in my hospital bed, I knew I would grab others by the hand and raise them up on a new limb...all so that I could tell them of the salvation of Jesus Christ and the grace of God that sustains me. Standing with Hope is more than just the name of the nonprofit organization I founded. It's a description of my life.[14]

Gracie and Peter, who is a pianist and composer, have performed for President George W. Bush as well as dozens of U.S. senators and governors. One of their most moving performances was the groundbreaking ceremony for the new amputee-training center for military personnel who have lost a limb.

No one would have blamed Gracie if she had become bitter and resentful about her lot in life. But Gracie's eyes sparkle, she's quick to laugh, and her smile lights up a room. That kind of beauty can't be found in an anti-aging serum; it comes from deep within. When you learn to handle adversity with grace, you become a poster child for the fountain of youth.

You can't package grace in a bottle. It's a gift God gives freely to those who ask for it, not something that can be bought over the counter. The apostle Paul begins most of his letters with the words, "Grace to you." Paul knew the value of grace and wished all his friends an abundance of it.

So how can you experience more grace in your life?

Be Gracious to Yourself

Do you beat yourself up over past mistakes? Do you replay scenes in your mind of your regrets and failures? I love the story my husband tells about a date that went wrong before he ever met me. He told his date a joke that bombed; she didn't even smile. After the date, he kept kicking himself for telling the joke. As he talked to his mom about it for the umpteenth time, she punched him in the arm.

"Ow. What was that for?" James asked.

"Stop beating yourself up about the date. You're making yourself miserable and starting to make me miserable too. It's over."

Can you relate? It's inevitable you'll make a mistake or two along the way. The question is how you deal with your failures. Learn from your mistakes, ask forgiveness of God and others if necessary, and move on. Give to yourself the grace you'd offer others. Remember the powerful words of Romans 8:1-2, "Therefore, there is now no condemnation for those who are in Christ Jesus, because through Christ Jesus the law of the Spirit of life set me free from the law of sin and death."

Be Gracious to Others

If you want to age prematurely, here's a formula to follow: criticize others, complain often, and regularly hold grudges. When we don't extend grace to others, we cut off the flow of God's grace into our own life. I'm thankful, on the other hand, that when we show grace to others, we open the door for all the blessings that accompany grace.

My mother is one of the most gracious women I know. She always sees the best in people and rarely speaks ill of anyone. As a result, she is well-loved and appreciated by her family, friends, clients, and community. As it says in Ecclesiastes 10:12, "Words from a wise man's mouth are gracious, but a fool is consumed by his own lips."

Need more grace in your life? Begin by giving it away.

BEAUTY TIP

To fill in the lines and imperfections of your face with grace, apply moisturizer with sunscreen or a makeup primer before putting on your makeup. This first layer will help create a smooth canvas and prevent foundation from caking into crevices.

Thought for Rejuvenation

Read this Scripture aloud from Isaiah 33:2,

> O LORD, be gracious to us;
> we long for you.
> Be our strength every morning,
>   our salvation in time of distress.

Now personalize it in prayer, "O Lord, be gracious to *me*; *I* long for You. Be *my* strength every morning, *my* salvation in time of distress."

Act of eXpression

Extend grace to each person you come in contact with today. If someone cuts you off on the road, resist the urge to blurt out, "Idiot driver!" If your coworker speaks rudely to you, chalk it up to a stressful day for her and pray for her.

Pluck Without Pain

Years ago when James and I were dating, we had a funny experience that could have ruined our relationship. James was unlike any man I'd ever met—an opinionated Italian from New York who was funny, godly, winsome, and totally unafraid to speak his mind. I adored him.

One evening we were sitting by the water's edge in Virginia Beach, Virginia. Holding hands, gazing into his eyes, I couldn't have been happier. Until he opened his mouth and said without any warning, "Arlene, have you ever thought of electrolysis?"

My mind was spinning. *What is electrolysis? How much does it cost? What part of my body needs it?*

Undaunted by my silence, he continued. "You have a few hairs above your lip, and just a few sessions of electrolysis will take that right off."

I wanted to hightail it to my car and hide my furry mustache as fast as I could. I was mortified. I have no idea what we talked about after that. All I could think was, *I have hair on my lip and he's staring at it.*

When I got home, I ran to the bathroom. Yep, James was right—I had a few dark hairs on my upper lip. I had never noticed those little hairs, but now I felt like Groucho Marx. I grabbed the phone book and started looking up electrolysis clinics. I learned electrolysis consists of inserting a thin metal device into the hair follicle and zapping it with a small amount of electricity. That didn't sound like much fun, but I was willing to try it once for love. I made my first appointment to get zapped for $50. After four treatments, my lip was hair free.

Losing the hair on my lip improved my appearance, boosted my confidence, and scored points with my future husband. Plucking unsightly things from our faces—whether it's lip hair or untamed eyebrows—is one way to look and feel younger.

In her book, *How Not to Look Old*, beauty expert Charla Krupp suggests you pluck your eyebrows after a bath or shower. The water plumps up hair, softens skin, and relaxes pores, so hairs come out easier. Or you can press a warm washcloth directly on your brow before tweezing.[15]

Pray First, Pluck Second

In a similar way, when you must pluck out of your life something much bigger than a hair follicle—such as a relationship or bad habit—you need to bathe it in prayer first for maximum results. Prayer acts as a buffer to make change easier and less painful. Follow these simple step-by-step instructions found in Philippians 4:6-7:

Step One: Do not be anxious about anything.

Step Two: But in everything, by prayer and petition, with thanksgiving, present your requests to God.

Step Three: And the peace of God, which transcends all understanding, will guard your hearts and minds in Christ Jesus.

When you pray first about the things you need to change in your life, God's peace will act as a supernatural pain killer, numbing you to the sting of transition. Is there anything you need to pluck out of your life to regain your youth and vitality? As you examine your heart, see if you can relate to any of these flaws that threaten the health of your spirit.

A Critical Spirit

Nothing saps joy and vitality like a critical spirit. Two ladies could be sitting next to each other in the same church service. One lady will walk away smiling and refreshed, thinking about all the things she learned and the wonderful people she spoke with. The other lady leaves annoyed, wondering when the pastor will ever come up with a decent sermon and why the people in the congregation are so shallow.

A critical spirit is an obsessive attitude of criticism and faultfinding. A woman with a critical spirit loves to complain and is usually upset about something. Unlike constructive criticism, which seeks to help others face-to-face, a critical spirit tears others down behind their backs. Locate a woman who is constantly judging and frowning, and you'll find a woman who looks ten years older than she really is.

A Comparing Spirit

I had the pleasure and pressure of going to graduate school with a handful of beauty pageant winners. It seemed in every communications class, I would meet a Miss California or Miss Pennsylvania. When I graduated from Regent University, I sat right next to Nicole Johnson, who would become Miss America in 1999. What about me? I wasn't Miss Anything.

It's easy to compare ourselves with others and come up short, isn't it? Measuring up to a beauty queen, triathlon winner, or successful CEO can be disheartening, to say the least. As our confidence plummets, so will our youth and vitality.

On the flip side, we can compare ourselves too favorably with others and think, "Thank God I don't look as bad as her." Puffing ourselves with pride will age us as well.

A Controlling Spirit

Have you ever known a control freak...or been one yourself? When someone has a controlling spirit, she desperately tries to dictate how everything around her is done. Clinical psychologist Les Parrott says, "Control Freaks are people who care more than you do about something and won't stop at being pushy to get their way."[16] Whether motivated by fear (something will go wrong if I don't intervene) or motivated by superiority (no one can handle this as well as I can), being a control freak is extremely taxing.

Do you wrestle with a critical, comparing, or controlling spirit? With God's help, you can pluck these damaging attitudes out of your life. Like having electrolysis, it may take more than one session, but if you're persistent in prayer, you will prevail with the help of the Holy Spirit.

HOW TO GET RID OF LIP OR CHIN HAIR

High-Cost Option: laser hair removal. Results are long lasting, but risks include burns and pain. Cost can be prohibitive; on average one area costs $200 and five to seven sessions are needed.

Medium-Cost Option: electrolysis or professional waxing. Cost for waxing the upper lip or chin is about $7 to $20 each.

Low-Cost Option: tweezing, home waxing, or shaving. These options cost less than $20 at any drugstore.

Thought for Rejuvenation

Can you identify with having a critical, comparing, or controlling spirit? If not, are there other character flaws you need to pluck out of your life?

Act of eXpression

Write down one way you can pluck out a character flaw in your life this week. Character flaw (for example, *a critical spirit*):

What I'm going to do differently this week (for example, *I will not say out loud the critical things I'm thinking in my mind*):

Day 8

Childlike Prayers

When my son was only four years old, to my delight he already had a tender heart for God. One night after bedtime prayers he said, "Mommy, I love God so much. I love Him from the top of our house to the bottom of the floor, then one billion inches down, and then back to the sky. That's how much I love Him. That's a lot. It's like 100 plus 50." After he said that, I ran to my computer to type it all down. It was a moment to capture and remember.

There's something very special about a young child praying to God. But come to think of it, you are a child of your heavenly Father. Is it possible to feel younger simply by praying like a child? How do you display childlike faith and perhaps unlearn some of those grown-up, stiff, predictable prayers? Here are a few things I've learned about childlike praying from my kids, Ethan and Noelle.

Pray with Enthusiasm

It's a common scene at breakfast. My kids Ethan, age five, and Noelle, age two, are seated around the table. I say, "Who wants to pray?" and both kids shout out "Me!" Their little hands shoot toward to the sky, urging me to pick them for this special distinction. I try my best to be fair and have them take turns, but regardless of who is chosen, both end up chiming in before the final amen. They are enthusiastic about prayer.

Now imagine you're at an adult prayer meeting at church. The pastor asks for volunteers to pray. Several seconds go by in silence. Finally, the woman in the third row who always volunteers lifts her hand. The rest of the congregation feels relieved that they don't have to pray out loud.

Whatever happened to that "pick me" enthusiasm? I'm not talking about being shy or outgoing; whether you pray aloud in public or alone in your room doesn't matter. The point is, when it's time to pray, do you think, *That's wonderful. Count me in.* Or do you sigh, *Okay, I guess I should.* To be childlike, you must pray with enthusiasm.

Come with Your Needs

I teach a Sunday school class for three-year-olds, and without fail, every week someone has a boo-boo to show off. Whether it's a skinned knee, ankle, or elbow, the story is the same: *Look at what happened to me. Will you pray it gets better?* When you're three years old, a boo-boo is a big deal, even if it happened a week ago and can barely be seen without a magnifying glass.

What are the needs—the cuts, the scrapes—in your life right now? Are there concerns weighing on your heart and mind? Come to God with your needs. He is waiting to give you comfort and healing. He's never too busy to hear about your boo-boos—no matter how big or small.

Be Persistent

For months my son has been praying about the same thing. Every night he ends his prayer with, "Help us to find #1 and #5. Amen." Those numbers refer to racecars he misplaced eons ago. Although I can't remember what they look like, he can, and he prays about them every single day. Ethan's prayer reminds me of Matthew 7:7-8, "Ask and it will be given to you; seek and you will find; knock and the door will be opened to you. For everyone who asks receives; he who seeks finds; and to him who knocks, the door will be opened." Be persistent in your prayers—ask, seek, knock—and God will answer you in due time.

Honest to Goodness

I love when kids pray because they are so brutally honest. Like this prayer found in a charming gift book called *Children's Letters to God*:

> Dear God,
>
> It rained for our whole vacation and is my father mad. He said some things about you that people are not supposed to say, but I hope you will not hurt him anyway.
>
> Your friend (but I am not going to tell you who I am)[17]

Isn't that funny? Take a cue from this anonymous boy or girl. Don't be afraid to be honest with your feelings, questions, confessions, and frustrations. God wants you to be completely honest—He can handle it.

Don't Forget to Say "Thank You"

Every parent wants their children to learn to say "please" and "thank you." Common courtesy applies in prayer too. It's not only polite to thank God for His many blessings; a heart of thanksgiving will keep you from becoming an old sourpuss.

I love a drama by my friend Paul Joiner titled "Treasured Prayers." Allow me to set the scene. It's Thanksgiving, and a single mom has invited her three grown children to share the holiday together. The three kids are irritated by their mother's attitude of thanksgiving despite her many hardships. They refuse to celebrate a holiday they don't believe in, and the conversation becomes tense and hostile. When her daughter declares God never helped them, the mother picks up a small wooden chest. Inside the chest are dozens of pieces of paper with writing on both sides.

The mother had written her prayer requests through the years for ice skates, asthma medicine, trips to Disneyland, and college scholarships. When each prayer was answered, she'd record the answer on the back. Her greatest treasure was this little humble wooden box filled with answered prayers.

Touched by their mother's faith, the children gather around their mom with a fresh understanding of how God had provided for them throughout their childhood. The drama ends with the mom saying that God had answered yet another prayer: that her children would come together to celebrate Thanksgiving as a family.[18]

Maybe it's time for you to begin a prayer box filled with your requests and then the answers as they come. Or you can list your needs in a journal and then check them off as God provides (don't forget to date them too). When you have a tangible reminder of the prayers God has answered, your faith will soar like a child's.

Add Seven Years to Your Life

Prayer is good not only for your soul; it's good for your physical health too. One article reports you can expect to live seven years longer if you nurture your soul through prayer, faith, and religious involvement. Studies have shown a strong correlation between heart health and religious faith. Praying patients who entered open-heart surgery were three times more likely to survive the surgery than people with no spiritual background.[19] Even if some in the medical profession compare prayer to a placebo, no one can argue with the benefits. Praying keeps you calm, provides peace during hard times, and gives a tremendous sense of hope.

Corrie ten Boom said it this way: "As a camel kneels before his master to have him remove his burden, so kneel and let the Master take your burden."[20] Why struggle with a heavy load of concern when you have a heavenly Father who offers to carry your burdens for you? First Peter 5:7 says, "Cast all your anxiety on him because he cares for you." Save your back, stay young, and hand over your heavy burdens to your Father in heaven.

Thought for Rejuvenation

Say this prayer out loud:

> Lord, I thank You for being my heavenly Father. I'm so glad You are always with me. I love You with all of my heart. Give me the faith and innocence of a child. Help me to trust in You more. I give my burdens and anxieties to You. Please help me with (name your specific concerns). Thank You for hearing and answering this prayer. Every good and perfect gift is from You. In Jesus' name, amen.

Act of eXpression

Begin a prayer journal or prayer box. Write down a prayer request and record how God answers.

Do What You Love

What did you dream of becoming when you were a teenager? Maybe you wanted to be a doctor, singer, actress, or homemaker. When you're young, it's second nature to dream of the things you want to do, the places you want to see, and the people you want to meet. But as you grow older, you understand a little better how the world works, and it's easy to lower your expectations. Sometimes the dreams of the past get buried in the demands of the present. You have bills to pay, obligations to your family and friends, and a long to-do list that never goes away. Doing what you love seems more like a luxury than a realistic goal.

Ask yourself this simple and clarifying question: Do you love your life and career (your career might be homemaking or retirement)? I'm not talking about a fantasy world where you love every single part of your job and enjoy every single minute of each day. Of course there will be aspects of your job you dread, and moments in many days when you wish you could go back to bed. But for the most part, do you love what you are doing right now?

Changing Careers After 50

When my friend Mary asked herself that question, the answer was no. I met Mary through my husband, who had the honor of being a personal business coach to Mary and her husband, Don. Mary is a cancer survivor, so she's one tough lady with a very tender heart. Before going into real estate, Mary and Don developed five long-term care facilities for the elderly. Years later those facilities were bought and staff was rearranged, so Mary and Don decided to take a big leap and venture into real estate.

Entrepreneurs by nature, they did very well with their new career as real estate agents. But Mary could never shake a nagging thought—she really missed working with the elderly and having an impact on families at such a personal level.

So after eight years of working in real estate, Mary took the plunge and made a career move in her fifties. She went back to work at the same assisted-living facility she left years earlier, and she loves it. Since it can be incredibly difficult to make a career move as you grow older, I asked Mary for some advice. She said, "I encourage someone to take her time because it's a big decision to leave a secure job and move to something different. But you do have to follow your passion. If you are passionate about what you do, it will work."[21]

Follow Your Passion

Because I'm five foot ten, I was constantly asked in high school if I played basketball. Although I had the height for it, I had absolutely no interest in basketball. Instead, I loved doing yearbook, student council, and cheerleading. I suppose I could have learned to play basketball, but it would have been short lived because my heart wasn't in it.

Maybe you're doing a job you're equipped to do, but you're not passionate about it. You *spend* time in the office, but you dream of *investing* time in something you really care about. Some days you feel like a ballerina on a football field. Do you want to make a career change, and if so, what's holding you back?

Barrier 1: I'm not qualified to do anything else.
Solution: Make a list of the skills you have mastered in your current job. You'll probably be surprised at the transferrable skills you already possess.

Barrier 2: I don't take risks.
Solution: Look before you leap. Research new opportunities thoroughly and interview people who are doing what you're interested in. If possible, shadow this person for a day to observe his or her routines. Don't quit your current job before securing a new job or having enough in savings to cover a few months of unemployment.

Barrier 3: I'm not an expert in the field I'm interested in.
Solution: Become an expert slowly but surely. If you are passionate about the subject, it will be enjoyable to learn more about your field of interest.

Check out books from the library, subscribe to related magazines, attend seminars, use the Internet, interview people in the field, and volunteer your time to learn more. Set aside time each day to expand your knowledge. Your perseverance will make you an expert, but it won't happen overnight.

Barrier 4: It's too late.

Solution: Remember, Mary was in her fifties when she changed careers. Valerie Ramsey, author of *Gracefully: Looking and Being Your Best at Any Age*, launched a career in modeling at age 63. It's never too late unless you decide it is.

Taking Stock

Maybe you don't have a clear picture of your ideal career, but you feel dissatisfied in your current role. Have you written a personal mission statement lately? A personal mission statement is a brief description of what you want to be and accomplish in your life. It's a tall order to formulate, but once you have something written down, it will make your decisions a lot easier. Having clear purpose in life is a huge factor in looking and feeling younger.

Stephen Covey said it well: "We don't invent our missions; we detect them."[22] Observe your attitudes and behavior during the week. What makes you feel alive and lights your fire? What bores you and saps your strength?

Hyrum Smith is the originator of the time-management system, the Franklin Planner. In his book, *What Matters Most: The Power of Living Your Values,* he shows readers how to discover what matters most and how to act on those values:

> Perhaps the most excruciating kind of pain comes from the gap—in some instances a wide chasm—between what we really value and what we are doing. This occurs when we realize that we are not living up to our potential or, even worse, that what we are doing doesn't match or is completely in opposition to what we really value, to what matters most to us…Wake up each morning and ask yourself, "What am I going to do today to close the gap between what I am doing and what really matters most to me?"[23]

Blowing Kisses

If you've ever visited Bermuda, you might be familiar with a man named Johnny Barnes. In 1983, Johnny was in his sixties, working as a driver and repairman at the bus depot. He got a crazy idea of how he could greet strangers and show them God's love. He stood at a roundabout in his hometown in Bermuda and began calling out to everyone he saw, "Good morning! God bless you!" People thought he was nuts, but morning after morning, he stood at that roundabout blowing kisses and smiling to commuters and pedestrians.

More than 25 years later, Johnny Barnes is still blowing kisses at that roundabout from roughly 3:45 a.m. to 10:00 a.m., five days a week. Today he is a legend and icon of hospitality in Bermuda. In a country where millionaires and billionaires are commonplace, Johnny Barnes is the only man honored with a statue in Bermuda. The 6½-foot tall bronze statue overlooks the entrance of East Broadway, honoring the simple man with the straw hat and infectious smile.[24] As a Christian, Johnny has prayed with countless people and shown the love of Christ in an unusual and memorable way.

Could you stand on a corner and blow kisses to strangers for six hours a day? Probably not, and that's okay. Johnny Barnes does it because he loves it. What would you love to do? (It's okay if it's a little crazy.)

Thought for Rejuvenation

Complete this sentence: Someday I'd like to...

Act of eXpression

Write a personal mission statement or read yours if you already have one. Here are a few questions to help you craft your mission statement:

- What do you imagine your life's mission to be about?
- If you knew you couldn't fail, what would you do?

- What are your natural talents and gifts?
- What do you love doing at work?
- What do you love doing in your personal life?
- Complete this sentence. I feel strongest when…

Begin your personal mission statement with words such as:

- I will…
- I can…
- I am…

My purpose is…

Your Personal Rx for the Mind

*Think positively about yourself, keep your thoughts and your
actions clean, ask God who made you to keep on remaking you.*

NORMAN VINCENT PEALE

Life is like a ten-speed bike; most of us have gears we never use.

CHARLES M. SCHULZ

It Starts with Your Sneakers

A few years after we were married, my husband and I went on our first European vacation to Italy and Switzerland. They say you can always tell who the Americans are by the shoes they're wearing. American tourists wear tennis shoes, and we were no exception. We walked and hiked through Zurich, Venice, Bellagio, and more wearing our unfashionable (but comfortable) sneakers, carrying our clothes and necessities in our backpacks.

One day, at beautiful Lake Como in Northern Italy, it poured down rain. We were soaked from head to toe and loved every minute of it (remember we were young). There was a space heater in our hotel room, so my husband placed his tennis shoes on the heater to dry. But his brilliant plan backfired because the heat popped the little air chambers in his Nike Airs. The next morning, instead of touring a glorious cathedral, we were asking directions to the nearest shoe store.

My husband has a strong aversion to flip-flops that was fueled by a train ride in Italy. Sitting in front of us was a teenage girl carrying a backpack that was about as big as she was. She wore flimsy flip-flops, and her feet were bloody, dirty, and all scuffed up. Clearly, those were the wrong shoes for her European vacation.

Flip-Flops or Tennis Shoes?

When you have an active lifestyle, you've got to be wearing the right shoes. No one works out at the gym in flip-flops or stilettos. If you're going to exercise, you've got to put on athletic shoes. So, how often do your tennis shoes get worn?

- Every day—I love the comfort.
- Several times a week when I exercise.
- I haven't laced up a pair of sneakers in weeks.
- I don't even know if I own tennis shoes.

If you have to go out and buy new tennis shoes because your old ones are worn out, that's a good sign—as long as it didn't take you ten years to wear them out. Owning a pair of good athletic shoes is one thing. Using them regularly for exercise is another.

Choose to Lace Up

Three times a week, my friend Jane wakes up at 5:00 a.m. to go walking with a friend. They walk outside if the weather permits, and work out indoors if it doesn't. Because there's no guesswork involved, they've been consistent in their exercise regimen for 18 years.

"I wouldn't wake up to exercise if there wasn't a knock on my door at 5:30 a.m.," Jane says. "It's a great idea to buddy up for exercise. We love to talk about the Bible while we walk and encourage each other."

Jane is reaping the numerous benefits of a healthy lifestyle. After she turned 65, she whispered to the receptionist at her doctor's office, "I have new insurance," because she didn't want to broadcast that she was now a card-carrying member of Medicare. Who could blame her—you can't tell by the way she looks.[1]

I'm sure there are mornings when Jane doesn't feel like getting up to welcome her friend. An active lifestyle doesn't begin with lacing up your tennis shoes; it begins with the *decision* to lace up those shoes. You must first make the choice to be healthy and active. Once you settle it in your brain—without question marks or excuses—the hard part is over.

Stick With the Schedule

Jane and her friend have been so successful with their walking because they treat their exercise time as a nonnegotiable appointment. Why is it that we can show up on time for a meeting, doctor's appointment, child's football game, or small group, but we're anything but prompt when it comes to exercise? Many women think of exercise as something to do during free time, but who has any free time anymore? We have to set aside time for the important matters of life, and exercise definitely qualifies.

If you're not used to exercising regularly, begin by reserving 30 minutes three times a week for exercise. Do not allow yourself to do anything else during that time. If you have unanswered phone messages or emails, just leave them alone. Your exercise time is not the time to put in a load of laundry or get dinner started. Guard those 30 minutes for exercise and exercise only.

Set a minimum amount of exercise per week and make sure you never dip below that minimum. Let's say you decide to exercise three times a week for 30 minutes each, and you get to the last day of the week and you haven't done a blessed thing. Guess that means you'll be taking a 45-minute walk in the morning and doing a 45-minute workout DVD that night to make up for the minutes you missed. Of course, many weeks you will exceed your minimum, and that's great.

Decide What to Do

Walking is a great exercise to begin with. Walk for 30 minutes around your neighborhood in the morning or in the early evening. Use that time to talk with the Lord, or invite a friend to buddy up with you. Walking can also be your default exercise if you can't think of anything else to do. Other ideas include:

- A home DVD workout
- Weight lifting at home with a pair of five- and ten-pound dumbbells
- Going to the gym—attend a class or make your own circuit
- Swimming
- Cycling
- Tennis
- Golf
- Dancing

My children's pediatrician is a woman in midlife who has more energy than a 25-year-old. She's thin, fit, and happy, with bright eyes and a chic haircut. Do you know what she does several times a week? Kickboxing. Just goes to show there are many ways to skin the cat of exercise—you just have to pick something you can enjoy with consistency.

I Feel Good

Once you win the battle and move from talking about exercise to actually doing it, something amazing will happen to your attitude. You'll have a sunnier outlook, more creative ideas, better problem-solving skills, and a calmer response to stressful situations. Exercise will make you feel good. In just a short time, you'll become addicted to your new exercise routine and feel more tired on the days when you don't work out. The more you recognize the immediate benefits of exercise, the more you'll want to exercise each week.

When I was pregnant in my late thirties, I felt blasé and lifeless in my first trimester. I dreamt of crawling under my blanket and staying there for several weeks. I didn't feel connected or passionate about anything. Because I felt so tired, my regular exercise regimen ceased. No one blamed me for my inactivity since pregnancy, like so many other medical conditions, was a great excuse.

About ten weeks into my pregnancy, I decided to go back to exercise class. I began once a week, riding a stationary bike. I found I was just as tired as before, so the exercise didn't wear me out further, but I felt so much better. My mood instantly lifted. The more I exercised, the more I felt like myself again. Exercise helped me emerge from my first-trimester funk.

Do you need to get out of an emotional funk? The surprising answer may be in your closet among your shoes.

Thought for Rejuvenation

"I discipline my body and keep it under control, lest after preaching to others, I myself should be disqualified" (1 Corinthians 9:27 ESV).

What are some specific ways you can discipline your body?

Act of eXpression

Take out your tennis shoes and use them at least three times to exercise within a week. If you don't own a good pair of athletic shoes, shop at an outlet or discount department store for a great deal.

Day 11

Brain Food

Yesterday, you were encouraged to regularly lace up your tennis shoes. A cute pair of athletic shoes will make you look and feel younger instantly. Plus, did you know exercise isn't just good for your emotional and physical health? It's great for your brain too. "The best advice I can give to keep your brain healthy and young is aerobic exercise," says Donald Stuss, PhD, a neuropsychologist and director of the Rotman Research Institute at Baycrest Centre for Geriatric Care in Toronto.[2]

Your brain cells, or neurons, have branch-like connections between them that are essential to thought. As you get older, these connections weaken. But brain research shows that exercise may slow down this mental decline. Aerobic exercise pumps more blood, nutrients, and oxygen into the brain, making for a healthier brain.

Studies by brain-health researcher Arthur Kramer at the University of Illinois have produced two significant findings: Fit people have sharper brains, and people who are out of shape but then get into shape sharpen their brains.[3] How exciting that exercise helps you not only fit into your skinny pants, it helps you remember where you stored those skinny pants in the first place.

Power Activities

Sadly, research shows that your brain starts slowing down at the young age of 30. But hold on, there's good news too. Several studies have shown that people of any age can train their brains to be faster, turning back the clock in their favor. The brain is a learning machine that responds positively to mental exercise. Neurologists say the brain is highly adaptable. If you ask it to learn something new, it will.

To keep your brain young, try any of these power activities:

- Learn a new language, instrument, or dance.

- Build a model airplane.

- Memorize a Bible verse and meditate on it throughout the day.

- Read a book that's completely different from what you typically read.

- Learn how to cook a new recipe.

- Do Sudoku, crossword, or jigsaw puzzles.

- Learn one new fact every day.

- Look up a new word in the dictionary.

- Find a problem in the newspaper and think about how you would solve it.

- Try doing things with your nondominant hand, such as opening the door or using keys.

- Use a different route to go to the grocery store.

- Memorize the words to a new song.

Memory-training specialist Harry Lorayne says in his book, *Ageless Memory: Simple Secrets for Keeping Your Brain Young,*

> Perhaps it's true that you can't teach old dogs new tricks. That's dogs, not people. I agree with Benjamin Franklin, who wrote, "No one is ever too old to learn." I try to learn something new every day. I sure tried to "learn something new" when I decided to get "involved" with computers when in my seventies. I was interested, enthusiastic to learn, and certainly curious to see what everyone was talking about. You need to set up some "mental push-ups."[4]

Have you been doing any mental push-ups lately? Like Harry Lorayne, are you interested, enthusiastic to learn, and curious about life? Maybe you want to learn, but you're wondering how to find the time for additional activities. Here's an easy tip: turn off the television. HGTV and the Food Network will go on without you. Instead of watching TV for even ten minutes, spend that time doing something that will feed your brain and keep it young.

Power Affirmations

It's important to challenge your brain with problems to solve and new things to learn, but it's also important to feed it a steady diet of positive affirmations. Olympic athlete Beverly Buffini (member of the 1988 U.S. volleyball team) has a simple and profound motto for her family of six children: "I Can, I Will, I Believe." I know from observing her that the motto is working as her children excel spiritually, academically, athletically, and socially.

If a sister could listen in to your thought life, what would she hear? Positive words of affirmation (*The best is yet to come*), or words of doom (*My life is over*). Your thoughts steer the direction of your life. Speaker and author Pam Farrel tells a story about Robin, her best friend and colleague in ministry:

> In midlife, it's easy to start complaining about aches and pains. Robin and her husband, Jack, have this rule. Anytime they're tempted to complain, they say "Think Young." They write "Think Young" in their calendar. It's posted in their house. Just having that little reminder to "Think Young" helps them decide to do things that are young. You don't want to put yourself in the old folks' home too early.[5]

Proverbs 23:7 says, "For as he thinks in his heart, so is he" (NKJV), so think young. Danna Demetre, RN and author of *Change Your Habits, Change Your Life*, says we change bad habits and adopt healthy habits through healthy mental programming. "It really starts with what we think about most often. If a woman of any age says, 'I can't stop eating. I hate to exercise,' her behavior will live out those lies."

On the other hand, when you speak words of life—"I love eating healthy food," and "My body is a temple of the Holy Spirit"—those affirmations will result in a positive change in your behavior.

Power Food

When you put a doughnut in your mouth, you might wonder about its impact on your waistline, but do you ever think about its effect on your brain? The same weight that slows you down as you climb the stairs also slows down your brain from making quick replies and witty comebacks. High blood pressure, diabetes, high cholesterol, and obesity all make life tough for the brain.

Colorful fruits, vegetables, beans, whole grains, nuts, spices, and (thankfully) dark chocolate contain antioxidants that are good for the brain. But there's another powerful nutrient that you may be lacking in your daily diet.

According to Danna Demetre, many women miss out on the benefits of an essential fatty acid called omega-3. Omega-3 fats stimulate the brain, revitalize the skin, slow down aging, improve fat metabolism, decrease inflammation, and protect your heart. Who wouldn't want to sign up for that? The best sources of omega-3 essential fatty acids are salmon, swordfish, tuna, shark, pecans, almonds, walnuts, soy nuts, flax seed, and deep green vegetables such as kale and turnip greens. But since most of us don't eat a serving of salmon every day, Demetre suggests supplementation:

> Many compelling studies are revealing that omega-3 supplementation decreases aggressive behavior, diminishes depression, protects against Alzheimer's disease, and fosters mental clarity. Just imagine your brain as healthy, well-nourished, and firing on all cylinders as opposed to undernourished like a car in bad need of a tune-up or needing a jumpstart to perform simple tasks. That jumpstart would be coffee and sugar, perhaps?[6]

Older Brain = Better Brain

To end on a positive note, older people are better at solving problems than young people because they have more mental history to draw from. There's a reason why the president of the United States must be 35 years of age or older, and why many people in their fifties and sixties are running the largest companies in America. As Barry Gordon, a neurologist at The Johns Hopkins School of Medicine and author of *Intelligent Memory: Improve the Memory That Makes You Smarter*, says, "It's nice to know some things get better with age."[7]

Thought for Rejuvenation

Make a list of things you like about your brain (for example, I am very good at remembering names; I am a great problem solver; I am creative):

Act of eXpression

Pick one Power Activity for the brain from today's reading and do it today.

4000 Hobbies

My friend Debbie had dreamt of going to Australia since she was ten years old. Growing up watching Jacques Cousteau on television, she wanted to see the Great Barrier Reef for herself. She planned to become an oceanographer until she saw a certain movie when she was 16. Can you guess what movie it was? *Jaws* may have changed her career path, but she always kept her love for the sea.

Decades later, Debbie was anticipating three milestones in her life: turning 50, celebrating 30 years at her job, and being a breast cancer survivor for 3 years. She wanted to celebrate in a meaningful way, so she decided to combine her passions—travel and photography—and plan an Australian adventure to the Great Barrier Reef. God provided every step of the way, from a free airline ticket using her frequent flyer miles to getting the last seat in the tour group she wanted. During this trip of a lifetime, she shot more than 2400 photographs and yes, finally swam in the Great Barrier Reef. About seeing the Great Barrier Reef, Debbie says, "I felt like I was on Cloud Nine. God loved me. I wasn't dead yet. I can't even describe the joy I felt."

Debbie's next adventure? Becoming a volunteer whaler on whale-watching cruises in her local city. She'll get to answer questions and share her love for the ocean with others. These hobbies and passions put the spring in Debbie's step and keep her young. She's constantly learning about things that interest her, plus she's excited about any opportunity to share Christ with the people she meets.[8]

The Adventurous Life

Pam Farrel writes about her adventurous friend, also named Debbie, in her book *Woman of Confidence*:

> She has hiked the Grand Canyon rim to rim and to the top of Yosemite's Half Dome alone. She biked across Europe several times. She has led seven trips to Russia to help with church planting and women's ministry. She has kayaked the Colorado River through the Grand Canyon. She took a ferry to Seward, Alaska, and then paddled back to Juneau on the open sea to her home on the backside of a glacier. In 2007 she was named the top outdoor educator in Alaska and was selected to lead the Discovery Channel team as they filmed their Alaskan specials.[9]

This woman has some serious hobbies. Like me, you may not have much in common with these adventurous Debbies. Your favorite hobby might be sitting in a lounge chair poolside, playing bridge, or bargain hunting at Nordstrom Rack. It doesn't matter *what* your hobby is; it just matters that you regularly do *something* you enjoy.

My mom loves cooking and arranging flowers. My sister-in-law Cindy enjoys glass blowing. My husband is learning how to play the guitar. We have longtime family friends who are retired doctors that enjoy dancing twice a week—the waltz, fox-trot, swing, and salsa. If you want to learn a new skill, such as dancing, playing an instrument, or knitting, check out your local community college. You'd be surprised at the wide offering of affordable classes ranging from sign language to woodworking for women.

Prayers and Squares

Sometimes you can even use your hobby to minister to others. When my friend Kay found out she had breast cancer, she received a prayer quilt from a group called "Prayers and Squares." This caring group of quilters sews unique quilts for cancer patients, sick babies, and people facing surgery or personal crisis. Before a quilt is given, the quilters tie knots in the quilt and pray for the recipient, literally blanketing them in prayer. "It had such an enormous impact on me," Kay says. Inspired by the quilt, she decided to begin quilting herself just three years ago when she was going through chemotherapy.

Kay started going to a quilting class at a continuing education center.

"The group totally embraced me. They were the most incredible women I had ever met. I was learning to quilt, and I got through breast cancer, radiation, and chemotherapy." Today, a healthy and vibrant Kay has started a "Prayer and Squares" group at her own church, giving back in a way that is both meaningful and fun.[10]

It's Never Too Late to Learn

If you were to see one of Kay's beautiful quilts, you would think she's been quilting for ages, but she's been doing it for only three years. She had a sewing background, which certainly helped, but she says sewing clothes and sewing quilts are vastly different. It just goes to show it's never too late to learn. It may not be as easy to pick up an instrument or learn a new language at age 65 compared to 5, but it can be done. You need one essential component: patience. New skills aren't attained overnight, but the perseverance required to learn will strengthen both your brain and your heart.

I love the story of Nola Ochs, who became the world's oldest college graduate at 95 when she received her diploma at Fort Hays State University in 2007. When she learned she was only 30 hours short of a bachelor's degree, she decided in her nineties to move 100 miles from her family farm to a university apartment to finish her degree. She earned a general studies degree with an emphasis in history, graduating alongside her 21-year-old granddaughter.[11]

If Nola Ochs can finish a college degree at 95, you can learn a new hobby at your current age. Neuroscientist Michael Merzenich, PhD, suggests keeping your brain young and healthy by doing activities that challenge and excite you: playing Ping-Pong, doing jigsaw or crossword puzzles, taking accordion lessons, mastering bonsai technique, or learning a new language. Merzenich says he has "4000 hobbies," which include a wood shop and a vineyard.[12]

You may not have 4000 hobbies, but do you have at least four? New adventures are waiting for you.

Thought for Rejuvenation

Make a list of four hobbies you enjoy. You can also include things you want to learn in the future.

Act of eXpression

Take out your calendar and schedule in time for one of the hobbies listed above. For example, if you wrote cycling, put a bike ride into your schedule in the next week. If you like cooking, sign up for a cooking class or buy yourself a new cookbook and try a few recipes this week.

Where Are My Keys?

My family and I were at the San Diego County Fair in search of the latest home improvement gadget. As we left one of the exhibit halls, my husband stopped abruptly.

"Where are my sunglasses?" he asked.

"On top of your head," replied a woman passing by.

"Thank you," my husband said, slightly embarrassed.

Another question my husband asks regularly is "Where are my keys?" I usually reply, "I don't know," or "I saw them in the bedroom," or "Why don't you just put them in the same place every day?" If it takes him more than a few minutes to find them, I usually join in the hunt. When the keys are found under a piece of mail or in the pocket of his pants, he teasingly blames me, as if I spend all my time concocting places to hide his keys.

Before you think women aren't as absentminded as men, allow me to confess something I misplaced that was far worse. I used to have this terrible habit of walking up to my car and placing my purse on the roof of the car while I opened the door. (Can you see where this is going?) One day, I got in my car, slammed the door shut, and drove away. When I got home, I realized my purse was gone and what I had done.

Someone had witnessed my purse fly from my car. He thought perhaps I had thrown the purse out of the car as a desperate attempt to get someone's attention, and so he made an effort to find it. Maybe this was the big clue to an abduction case. He took the purse home, figured out my phone number, and called. It wasn't a kidnapping after all, just a brainless blunder by a perfectly safe woman.

Losin' It

Do you ever go through your day and wonder, *Where is my head?* Maybe you can't find your keys, bills, or favorite necklace. Or maybe you've misplaced something big like a purse. As you grow older, you can feel more forgetful. But many times age has very little to do with your frustration about finding things. Your problem isn't a memory issue; it's an organizational issue. Surrounded by too much stuff, it's easy to think, *I'm losing my mind*. But Marcia Ramsland, author of *Simplify Your Life*, says, "It's important to realize you're not losing your mind. Your system is broken. It's not a character flaw or an age issue. It just means you're handling more things and you need to create systems to deal with the changes in your life."[13]

What kind of systems work? Marcia uses the acronym PUSH to help women simplify their lives.

P is for Project—A one-time focused investment to simplify an area of life

U is for You—You've got to organize in a way that makes sense to you

S is for System—Create a dependable plan that maintains the project you just completed

H is for Habit—A valuable personal daily routine to stay organized[14]

After interviewing Marcia about organization, I was convicted, motivated, and then empowered to do something with all my piles of junk around the house. It was time for a PUSH. I went to work on the clutter in the family room and ended up with three bags of stuff to give away. It felt great.

Use It or Lose It

As we get older, we accumulate more things from each season of life: college yearbooks, binders from various seminars, training manuals, awards, photographs, sentimental gifts, and much more. According to Marcia, the key isn't just organizing your stuff—it's being able to simplify and let go of things from the past you don't need. I love her simple adage, "Use it or lose it."

But what if you're a pack rat or treasure hunter? What if you can't bear to part with that ticket stub from ten years ago, the rock collection your son once held dear, and the dress you wore to your high school prom? Keep repeating Marcia's adage, "Use it or lose it." Take pictures of your beloved items before you toss them or give them away. Here are three specific examples to help you get started:

1. After teaching organization for more than 24 years, Marcia had accumulated a lot of paper. She handed her son four inches of paper, and he returned 20 minutes later with all of those papers scanned onto a small flash drive. So far, she's gotten rid of 66 pounds of paper in her files by scanning them and keeping them electronically.

2. Wondering how to sort all your jewelry? Look at your current jewelry area and ask yourself, "What would I like my jewelry drawer to look like so I can get dressed quickly?" Maybe this means putting your everyday favorites in a jewelry box and putting the rest of your collection in a shoebox. Whatever doesn't fit in the shoebox is given away. If your jewelry has sentimental value, take a picture of it before saying goodbye.

3. Are your bookshelves sagging with too many books? When Marcia had to move, she realized how expensive it would be to pack all her books since she was paying by the pound. Her library contained 440 titles; she decided to pare that down by 50 percent and gave away 220 titles. Instead of mourning the loss of all those great books, she created a goal to strive for and felt wonderfully satisfied when she achieved it. Plus she thought of those books blessing someone else who would read them.[15]

Getting Started

Simply reading about getting organized isn't going to magically turn your house around, but it is a start. Your next step is to get rid of clutter and put systems of organization into place that will work long-term for you and your family. The first area to tackle is your kitchen and family room since you likely spend the most time in those places. Begin by putting things away after every meal and eliminating the clutter in the family room that hasn't been touched in ages, such as old magazines or newspapers.

About those troublesome keys, take the advice of Karen Ehman, author of *The Complete Guide to Getting and Staying Organized*, and have one special place for your keys. Karen's keys are always in one of two places: in the ignition or hooked to her purse. I had to ask if she ever misplaces her purse, but she has a particular place for that too. Karen says,

> If you don't have a plan for where your keys go (or whatever item), you're just going to set them down wherever it's convenient and then you can't remember where you put them. For me it's helpful to free up brain space and put them in the same place. Being organized boils down to being prepared.[16]

Are you ready to free up some of that needed brain space?

Thought for Rejuvenation

Do you ever feel as if you're losing your mind because you can't find something? List three specific areas in your home that frustrate you the most.

1.

2.

3.

Act of eXpression

Take one of those areas and spend 15 minutes today decluttering that area. Brainstorm a way to make that area easier to organize for you.

Whatever Happens, Remain Calm

I have never liked getting a foot massage. It tickles! But James loves them. When we were dating, he would ask me to take my shoes and socks off so he could massage my feet. I thought that was horrendous. First of all, I didn't want him smelling my stinky feet. Then, I certainly didn't want him touching them. It was torture by tickling. I tried to avoid his requests as much as possible, and it wasn't until we were married that I realized why he kept offering to rub my feet. He wanted me to massage *his* feet in return. That never dawned on me. "Do unto others" meant I would never touch his feet because I didn't want mine touched. To James, "Do unto others" meant, "If I massage her feet, someday she'll return the favor."

Now that we're married, he doesn't try to massage my feet, and I'm happy to massage his. After a stressful day, a five-minute foot massage seems to work wonders for James. Doing something you find relaxing has many benefits, including lower blood pressure, improved cardiovascular health, and a better night's sleep.

Do you set aside a few minutes each day to relax and allow yourself to calm down? Part of staying young is your ability to remain calm, no matter what life throws you. You've certainly seen the opposite—the woman who nervously goes through life, always stressed or worried about something that's hanging over her head. Too much stress not only strips your soul of peace; it causes all sorts of problems for your mind and body.

Research shows that stress hormones such as cortisol block weight loss. When you're stressed, your body interprets that as a type of famine and hoards all the fat it can. Stress is also hard on the brain, interrupting healthy processes such as learning or memory.[17] For instance, one area of your brain called the hippocampus is responsible for memory. Chronic stress weakens the hippocampus; no wonder you feel scatterbrained when you're really stressed.

So how can you combat stress in your life? Try engaging every day in relaxing rituals that are meaningful to you. Exercise is always a great de-stressor, whether you're walking, stretching, or weight lifting. Meditating on God's Word will calm the fiercest of storms. I know that Proverbs 3:5-6 served as an anchor for me during a tumultuous time.

Trust in the Lord Even When

When I was 20-weeks pregnant with my second child, I read a devotional from Proverbs 3:5-6, a familiar and favorite passage:

> Trust in the LORD with all your heart
>> and lean not on your own understanding;
> in all your ways acknowledge him,
>> and he will make your paths straight.

I felt the Lord tug on my heart, "Hang on to this verse today. It's special for you." That day was the highly anticipated ultrasound date when James and I would find out if we were having a boy or a girl. My in-laws were visiting from out of town for Thanksgiving, and the mood was festive—until we were in the radiology office. The ultrasound technician was very serious, somewhat of a killjoy, and strangely quiet. We found out we were having a girl and were sent home.

A few hours later, my doctor called. "Arlene, I hate to tell you this, but your baby has serious chromosomal defects and she isn't going to make it. She will probably die in the womb in the next few days. I'd really like you to go to the specialist today for a detailed ultrasound so you don't have to go through the entire Thanksgiving weekend not knowing."

I never imagined hearing those words, but a wave of peace came over me. *Trust in the LORD...* The specialist confirmed that my baby's heart would stop beating within days, maybe one to two weeks at the most. That was very hard news to hear the day before Thanksgiving. I struggled with what I should say when acquaintances asked about the baby. At church that weekend, I went forward for prayer and found great comfort in my sorrow. God had always been faithful to me in the past; certainly He would be faithful now. *Trust in the LORD…*

One week went by, and then another, and my little girl's heart kept on beating. In my prayers, I asked God for one of three things:

1. Take my baby home to be with You.

2. Heal my baby.

3. Give us grace to raise a baby with special needs.

The hardest part was waiting. What would happen to our family? Six weeks later, her heart was still beating, to the doctor's amazement. She was still with us on Christmas Day. But a few days later, she was gone.

Unfortunately, the story didn't end there. I still had to deliver that precious baby. *Trust in the LORD…* The day I was scheduled to be induced, I started labor naturally. It was a physically and emotionally difficult delivery, but God's presence was thick in that hospital room. I knew God was watching over me, singing words of comfort while I labored for a child that had been lost.

I never saw that little girl, who we named Angel Rose. The doctor suggested it would be better not to see her, and we agreed. But my family did receive a photograph of her feet, and her tiny footprints in clay. Those have become the most precious reminders of God's nearness during our time of brokenness.

We held a memorial service at the beach for Angel Rose with a few close friends and family members. I read a letter to her and said goodbye. Our eyes gazed up at the blue sky as a bouquet of balloons rose to the heavens, a visual reminder of our little girl's new home.

I can honestly say my memories of Angel Rose are all sweet. In her short life, she taught me to trust in God as I never have before. She taught me to be thankful for each day of life. On what would have been her due date, I took a pregnancy test and it was positive. Nine months later, I gave birth to a healthy girl named Noelle Joy. The previous Christmas I said goodbye to a little girl, and just one Christmas later, I was holding another in my arms. *Trust in the LORD…*

Since that time, God has used Angel Rose's story to encourage many moms who have experienced miscarriage and stillbirth. I even had the opportunity to share Angel's story on *The Hour of Power* with Dr. Robert Schuller.[18] It just goes to show God stands ready to use your darkest times as a testimony of His ability to give supernatural grace, if you'll let Him.

If you need help during stressful times, cry out to God and He will deliver you. Take a few minutes daily in prayer or by listening to your favorite worship music to let go of your stress. It's easy to remain calm, no matter what happens, when you know God is on your side.

Thought for Rejuvenation

Meditate on Philippians 4:6-7, "Do not be anxious about anything, but in everything, by prayer and petition, with thanksgiving, present your requests to God. And the peace of God, which transcends all understanding, will guard your hearts and your minds in Christ Jesus."

Act of eXpression

What is something that calms you down? A walk around the block? A massage? Soft music? Prayer? Reading? Playing the piano? Journaling? Set aside five minutes today to do something relaxing for yourself.

Day 15

Laugh and Eat Chocolate

I had always dreamed of a fairy-tale wedding complete with the perfect dress, ceremony, and groom. Well, my dream almost came true.

The morning of the wedding, my hairdresser said, "Sweetie, today is your wedding day. Something is bound to go wrong. It always does. Whatever happens, just enjoy it and laugh, because it's your special day."

The ceremony began right on cue. My aunt, a polished pianist, was playing the piano beautifully. The families had been seated. I was standing in the foyer, holding my father's arm. The bridesmaids were lined up in front of me. Then something alarming happened.

Dr. Charles Holman, one my husband's favorite seminary professors, was officiating the wedding. When the music stopped briefly—it was about to change for the bridesmaids to enter—Dr. Holman took that as his cue to begin the ceremony.

"Dearly beloved, we are gathered here in the sight of God and man to bring together James and Arlene in holy matrimony." The only problem was I was still in the hallway. He continued for what seemed an eternity reading his notes, never noticing that I (the bride, the star of the show) had not even entered the building. Finally, he asked, "Who gives this woman to this man in holy matrimony?" Baffled, he looked for my father to answer the question and realized he had begun without us.

Meanwhile, out in the foyer, I was incredulous and in need of some oxygen. Who would have ever imagined I'd miss the beginning of my own wedding? The doors opened, and those bridesmaids flew down the center aisle. My moment to enter had finally arrived.

You could feel the tension lift out of the church as I walked down that aisle. Dr. Holman recovered beautifully, making a joke of his terrible mistake and conducting the rest of the ceremony with warmth, sincerity, and no further foibles.

I remembered the advice of my hairdresser just hours before. *Something is bound to go wrong. It always does.* Yes, something big had indeed gone wrong, but you know what? I didn't mind having my "picture perfect ceremony" ruined. Quite the contrary, I couldn't have planned a more memorable, funny, unpredictable, priceless moment.

Funny Failures

When things don't turn out exactly as you planned, learn to laugh. Isn't it true that the funniest things happen when life doesn't go according to the script? That's probably why *America's Funniest Home Videos* is still airing after 19 seasons. Viewers keep tuning in to watch funny accidents, mishaps, and practical jokes. Bumps, bruises, and broken items are funny when they happen to someone else. They're much harder to laugh about when they happen to you.

If you can learn to laugh despite the many inconveniences life throws your way, you'll be able to stay young longer. You can even poke fun at the aging process as Pam Farrel does in her book, *Fantastic After 40: The Savvy Woman's Guide to Her Best Season of Life:*

> *Old Is When*
> Going braless pulls all the wrinkles out of your face.
> Getting lucky means you find your car in the parking lot.
> An all-nighter means not getting up to use the bathroom.[19]

Laughter Is Good Medicine

There's good reason why television sitcoms, funny movies, and comedy acts are popular. It feels good to laugh. Even the medical community attests to the positive power of laughter. Studies have shown that laughter increases dopamine, which is the pleasure chemical messenger in the brain. Laughing gives your face a break since it takes five times as many muscles to frown. Your lungs get a good workout during a belly laugh, providing more oxygen for the body. Laughing helps your abs too, and compared to sit-ups, it's a lot more fun. Laughter can also act as a natural painkiller, increasing your tolerance for pain.

In his 1979 book, *Anatomy of an Illness,* Norman Cousins describes how he fought the pain of a prolonged illness with laughter. He checked into a hotel room and put himself on an unorthodox dose of vitamins, funny books, and movies. His symptoms ceased.[20] Over the years, researchers have explored the impact of laughter and health. They've found that laughter can help you cope with stress, strengthen your immune system, decrease pain, and even reduce your risk of heart disease.

British researchers tested a group of men and women, ages 35 to 55, to measure how many happy moments they had throughout the day. They found the happiest people had 32 percent lower levels of the stress hormone cortisol, which has been linked to abdominal obesity, type 2 diabetes, high blood pressure, and other disorders. The happy group also had lower levels of fibrinogen, an inflammatory marker that predicts future coronary heart disease. On the other hand, the least-happy people in the study had 12 times higher levels of this problematic chemical.[21]

Ha-Ha-Ha

Maybe you'd like to have more laughter in your life, but you just don't think of yourself as a funny person, or there's not much to laugh about in your life right now. You can glean some tips from "Laughter Clubs," a unique social experience offered at retirement homes, therapists' offices, and medical centers such as the Cancer Treatment Center of America.

If you were to walk into a Laughter Club, first there's the greeting laugh. You make eye contact with another person in the laughter club and start belly laughing. Sure, it's contrived at first, but it's not long before genuine laughter kicks into gear. And even if it doesn't, fake laughter has been documented to have positive effects as well.

Then the group leader takes the participants through laugh-related exercises. In one exercise, all the participants stand in a circle with the leader in the middle. Each person puts their fingertips on their cheekbones, chest, or lower abdomen and makes "ha ha" sounds until they feel vibrations in their body. Before long, everyone is laughing because laughter is contagious.

You can create your own laughter club at home by greeting your family members with a smile and laugh, watching a funny home movie or favorite sitcom after dinner, or playing charades to depict how your day went.

Divine Dark Chocolate

Chocolate also alleviates pain. My grandmother lives in an assisted living center, and I bring her one pound of assorted dark chocolates whenever I visit. She looks forward to it and so do I because she shares. Thankfully, research is on the side of dark chocolate, praising the antioxidants found in dark chocolate that contains over 70 percent cocoa.

I love how this WebMD article, "Dark Chocolate Is Healthy Chocolate," begins: "Got high blood pressure? Try a truffle. Worried about heart disease? Buy a bon-bon."[22]

That's the kind of health advice women like. But before you go chocolate crazy, remember you still have to deal with the extra calories of that dark chocolate bar, so think moderation. I remember buying a one-pound dark chocolate bar that I was going to use for baking at Christmastime. I got busy and didn't bake a thing. I hate to admit I ate that giant bar instead—not in one sitting, but let's say it didn't take me much longer than that.

See, there's a funny failure I can laugh about (and not repeat anytime soon, I hope).

Thought for Rejuvenation

How often do you laugh per day?

☐ I'm lucky if I crack a smile

☐ One to ten times

☐ Ten to twenty times

☐ Too many times to count

Act of eXpression

Create your own laughter club this week. Watch an episode of a favorite funny show. Skip the front page of the newspaper and read the comics instead. Look through an old family album and retell your favorite funny stories.

Day 16

What's Next?

You've heard of "death by chocolate," but have you ever heard of "death by destination"? It's a phrase I like to use to represent what happens when you arrive at a goal, only to stop growing. It happens when you've reached the top of the corporate ladder and you switch on the cruise control. It happens when you feel stuck in your circumstances and ambivalent about the future. It happens when your kids are grown and gone, and you find yourself staring at an empty calendar.

Empty Nest, Empty Schedule

Marcia Ramsland remembers when her youngest child graduated from college and all three of her children were out of the house. For 28 years, she poured her heart and soul into parenting. She had achieved her life goals: raising her children and publishing her book, *Simplify Your Life: Get Organized and Stay That Way.* She wondered what was next. Have you ever wondered the same thing?

Marcia decided to give the rest of her days to the Lord. An organizer by nature, she couldn't imagine what a 20- or 30-year plan would look like. She decided to focus on something until her next zero birthday, which happened to be 60. Her strength is speaking and writing, so she told the Lord she would speak wherever He wanted.

After that prayer, the Lord uprooted her and her husband from San Diego to Dallas. In Dallas, she got involved in a group called Women in Christian Media, wrote a second book, organized a large church staff, and began speaking at Lifestyles Conferences. God had taken her prayer seriously and was using her to speak and write. But to her surprise, within 14 months, she was headed back to San Diego.

Happy to be back, Marcia helped establish a Women in Christian Media group on the West Coast, plus she continues to write books and speak. But like most of us, Marcia experiences seasons when there are more opportunities than minutes in the day, and then other seasons, when nothing seems to be happening at all. Marcia says,

> Whenever you're in a lull in life ask yourself, What do I need to do to get ready so if someone called up and said "I want you to write a book, you're going to be on *Oprah*, or I want you to take a six-month sabbatical," you would say, "Okay, I'm ready" because you have prepared in the in-between time of life. That's what it's all about, following the Lord every day and saying, "Here's my life, what's next?"[23]

Women have so many opportunities that Marcia encourages women to take time each September to ask a simple question: *Do I want to be doing this same thing next year?* If the answer is no, then begin making changes in your career or activities to reflect your heart's desire. Add new activities to your life, hang around young people, and pour into younger women coming up behind you. In so doing, Marcia says your energy will be revitalized.[24]

Lessons from the Anchor Desk

Television news is a tough business characterized by turnover, yet veteran anchor Carol LeBeau managed to stay at one station in San Diego for 28 years. After anchoring the news for ABC affiliate KGTV, Carol turned in her press pass for retirement. As you can imagine, there were days when the transition was tough.

"People point to me in public and say, 'Ooh, lady on the news,'" LeBeau says. "They can't think of my name, but they know I'm the lady on the news. I'm not the lady on the news anymore."

The week after her retirement, Carol was emceeing an event where she was asked to introduce herself. For the first time in decades, she didn't know what to say. She ended up saying to the crowd, "I used to work at Channel 10 news, but I guess for tonight I am a child of God and the proud wife of a retired Navy pilot."

Shortly afterward, Carol had orthopedic surgery, so in a matter of months she was stripped of two things she once found her identity in: her position and physical fitness. As a strong believer in Christ, Carol has held on to the Scripture that's engraved on her bracelet, "Lo, I am with you always." She says,

> It doesn't matter what your transition, other people have gone through it before you. If you can talk yourself down from the ledge and say, "Wait a minute. Are you going to be the first person in the universe to work at a job for 400 years or have kids that don't grow up and start their own families?" No. This is part of the cycle of life. The notion that the world isn't going to spin on its axis without me is foolish, prideful, and just plain silly. You've got to be open to God for what He has next.[25]

Setting New Goals

Olympic athlete and mother of six, Beverly Buffini, knows a lot about moving toward new goals. She writes in her book, *I Can, I Will, I Believe*:

> Set goals for yourself and write them down on paper. I have witnessed and experienced first-hand the startling effectiveness of this simple procedure. Make your goals realistic and reachable, but not necessarily small. I will teach my children how significant it is to set goals, and I will encourage them to keep their sights on their GREAT BIG AUDACIOUS GOALS. But I will also make sure they know that true wealth or success in life is found along the way…The reward comes in searching and expecting and working hard at it, as if trying to find a hidden treasure.[26]

The Christian life should be characterized by a zeal for good works and personal growth. Don't be content to sit on the sidelines because you feel your best days are behind you. Keep pressing forward and allow the Holy Spirit to give you power for fresh creation instead of falling asleep on the bench. Ulrich Zwingli, the leader of the Protestant Reformation in Switzerland, said, "Our confidence in Christ does not make us lazy, negligent, or careless; but on the contrary, it awakens us, urges us on, and makes us active in living righteous lives and doing good."[27]

Are you ready for whatever God has for you next?

Thought for Rejuvenation

Imagine it's your ninetieth birthday. What kind of tribute would you like to hear? What accomplishments do you want mentioned? What character traits do you want to be known for?

Act of eXpression

What might the next step be for you? Do one thing this week to prepare yourself for this new challenge or activity.

Your Personal Rx for the Body

To lengthen thy life, lessen thy meals.
BENJAMIN FRANKLIN

A bear, however hard he tries,
grows tubby without exercise.
WINNIE THE POOH

Day 17

Plastic Surgery, Botox, and Other Modern Marvels

Some celebrities would like to conceal their facelifts, but comedian Phyllis Diller was never one of them. Her one-liners about plastic surgery brought her fame and endeared her to women and plastic surgeons alike. Punch lines like:

"The only parts left of my original body are my elbows."

"My Playtex Living Bra died...of starvation. I never made Who's Who, but I'm featured in What's That?"

Phyllis Diller talked openly about cosmetic surgery decades before it was common to do so. The American Academy of Cosmetic Surgery even presented Diller with its first annual Franklin Ashley Award, given to her for advancing the acceptance of cosmetic surgery.[1]

Today cosmetic surgery has gone mainstream. You can redefine your nose with rhinoplasty, bring out your cheeks with facial implants, enlarge or reduce your breasts, tighten up your tummy, or smooth out your wrinkles with Botox. Between 1996 and 2000 the number of cosmetic procedures more than doubled, growing from one to three million per year in the U.S.[2] But this boon in plastic surgery isn't all good news. Many women have been stuck with unrealistic expectations, unqualified surgeons, and unpaid surgical bills.

Unrealistic Expectations

Having cosmetic surgery will change your appearance, but it won't change your life. Too many women think, *If only I could get rid of the cellulite on my thighs, then I would be happy.* Thinner thighs may bring temporary pleasure, but it's just a matter of time before life continues as before. The communication problems with your spouse or children will still exist. Your coworker will still have that annoying habit. You'll still be tempted to eat too much chocolate cake. If you're banking on some plastic surgery to radically improve your life, you're setting yourself up for some serious disappointment.

I think of a scene from the 1993 movie *Cool Runnings* about a ragtag group of athletes who form the highly laughable Jamaican bobsled team at the 1988 Olympic Winter Games. Their coach, a fictional character played by John Candy, had a dishonorable past. He had lost his gold medal in a previous Olympics when he was caught putting extra weights in his team's bobsled. The night before the Jamaican team's Olympic race, one of the bobsledders, Derice, talks to the coach about his desire for a gold medal.

> *Coach:* Derice, a gold medal is a wonderful thing. But if you're not enough without one, you'll never be enough with one. [*Turns to leave.*]
>
> *Derice:* Hey coach, how will I know if I'm enough?
>
> *Coach:* When you cross that finish line tomorrow, you'll know.

Friend, if you're not enough without plastic surgery, you'll never be enough with it. You were lovingly and beautifully created by God. If you feel insecure about your appearance, the true transformation of beauty will first happen in your mind and heart, not on the surgery table.

Unqualified Surgeons

As the demand for plastic surgery has grown dramatically, more and more procedures are performed by doctors with little training in this area. In the past, cosmetic surgery was primarily done by plastic surgeons. Now many physicians have entered the profitable cosmetic surgery field, and in most states, no law prevents physicians to advertise as plastic surgeons, even if they have no training in plastic surgery.

When looking for a qualified plastic surgeon, ask if the surgeon is certified by the American Board of Plastic Surgery (ABPS). There's a big difference between "board certified" and "certified by the American Board of Plastic Surgery," which has rigorous requirements. Other boards may sound impressive, but requirements may be minimal. Some boards have even been accused of existing solely to give credibility to their members.

Unpaid Surgical Bills

Cosmetic surgery isn't cheap, and if you choose to finance your procedure, you may be paying for your nip and tuck for months. Here are the average costs of popular procedures:

- Botox injection—$500

- Breast augmentation—$6,000

- Facelift—$8,000

- Forehead lift—$4,000

- Liposuction—$3,200

- Rhinoplasty (nose surgery)—$5,000

- Tummy tuck—$6,500

Botox Beauties

I've shared a few precautions about cosmetic surgery. On the flip side, many women have tried cosmetic surgery and loved it. Recently I was sitting next to a sharp, energetic, hip lady on an airplane. We started chatting, and I discovered she had already attended her forty-fifth high school reunion. It didn't seem possible since she looked so young. She smiled broadly and said with a twinkle in her eye, "Yes, I did look much better than many of my friends." In addition to her love for life and good taste, she's had a Botox injection or two.

Since 1997, plastic surgeons have been using Botox injections to improve or eliminate facial wrinkles. Botox, which is derived from the same bacteria that causes botulism, can be injected by your plastic surgeon to eliminate crow's feet, frown lines, and forehead wrinkles. These wrinkles are caused by repetitive facial expressions.

So if you constantly raise your eyebrows, you're going to get more wrinkles on your forehead. If you squint, pout, purse your lips, or wrinkle up your nose as a habit, you'll get wrinkles faster in those areas. Ask a spouse or a friend to observe your facial expressions. I just noticed that my husband raises one eyebrow and his forehead wrinkles when he takes a drink of water. Is there something you constantly do? Look at yourself in the mirror as you recreate some of your most used facial expressions. You can minimize wrinkles simply by retraining yourself to use body language that doesn't produce lines on your face.

If you choose to use Botox, plastic surgeons say you will see improvement within 24 hours and continue to see improvement in your wrinkles for one week. Botox is most effective for the forehead and frown lines between eyebrows (notice there are no lines there when you smile). Results last for about two to twelve months, with the average duration being four to six months.

To learn more about the risks and benefits of plastic surgery, talk to your friends who have had similar procedures, read books from the library on the subject, and interview plastic surgeons if you're really interested. Do your homework before you decide on any procedure. Like they say in woodworking, "Measure twice, cut once."

TIP FOR CONTACT LENS WEARERS

Every time you put in or take out your lenses, most likely you're pulling open the skin around your eye. Since that skin is delicate, try removing your contact lens without pulling on the skin above and below your eye. Just put your clean fingertips on your lens and pull straight out without disturbing your skin.

Thought for Rejuvenation

Are there any areas on your face or body that you wish you could change? List them here:

What could you improve without cosmetic surgery?

Act of eXpression

Have a spouse or close friend observe your facial expressions throughout one day. Have him or her tell you when you do something that causes wrinkles, such as pouting or scrunching up your face. Chances are you're not even aware of it. Look at yourself in the mirror making those expressions, and then make a conscious effort to limit those wrinkle-producing expressions.

I'm Not 13, But My Hormones Are Raging!

Do you remember your first period? I don't remember mine very well, so I suppose it wasn't too traumatic. I recently saw a trendy kit to help teenage girls prepare for that first period. The kit included a question and answer booklet, a calendar to track her periods, pads, panty liners, and wipes, all packaged in a cute pink bag. The kit is meant to help a girl celebrate this rite of passage into womanhood. Next, maybe someone should create a menopause kit to celebrate that rite of passage, complete with a handheld fan, bottle of chilled water, and dark chocolate.

You may not be 13 anymore, but your hormones are raging. Your mood swings up and down with the slightest provocation, you're teary-eyed and emotional during commercials, and your nights are hot—not with sex but with hot flashes. Who has taken over your body, and when are they going to give it back?

First there's perimenopause, a transition into menopause that happens years before menopause when your ovaries produce less estrogen. Perimenopause usually begins in a woman's forties, but can start as early as the thirties. Signs of perimenopause include hot flashes, breast tenderness, worsening of PMS, lower sex drive, tiredness, irregular periods, and difficulty sleeping. For some, perimenopause may come and go with little fanfare over a few months. For others, it may last for years.

Then comes menopause, when you stop having your period, which sounds like a great deal until you realize you may be swapping menstruation for insomnia, mood swings, depression, irritability, fatigue, decreased libido, and hot flashes. The average age of menopause is 51, with hot flashes taking center stage for the most common and irritating symptom. Two-thirds of women in America complain of hot flashes during peri-menopause, and most women deal with hot flashes at some point during menopause.[3]

Turn Down the Heat

When Danna Demetre, popular speaker, RN, and author of *The Menopause Guide*, hit 50, her emotions went topsy-turvy. She used to tell her husband, "You can get away from me. I'm stuck in here." She began getting outrageous hot flashes at night. At first, she'd wake up once a night, then twice, then three times. Does this sound familiar? About 75 percent of menopausal women suffer hot flashes. Nighttime hot flashes are more common, resulting in chronic sleep deprivation, a recipe for disaster for the midlife woman with enough stress on her shoulders already.

"The ceiling fan running all night long has saved me," Danna said. "That's a little thing, but it truly makes a difference." Danna encourages women to ask: Is it time to try herbal supplements or hormone replacement, or am I just going to stick it out? For Danna, since the hot flashes disrupted her sleep for many months, she made the choice to move from herbal supplements to bioidentical hormones. Her doctor's philosophy was to make it natural and to take the lowest dose possible for the shortest amount of time. Over the course of five years, Danna dropped the dose three times until it was very low, and then she never went above that dose again.[4]

Hot flashes vary from woman to woman. Some women have hot flashes for a short time, while others wonder when the constant heat will ever simmer down. Generally, hot flashes are less severe as time passes. My mother-in-law swears by the power of the swimming pool. She says there's nothing like submerging yourself under that cool water to keep hot flashes at bay. On the flip side, avoid Jacuzzis and hot showers like the plague. Other things you can do include:

Keep your bedroom cool at night. Get a ceiling fan or other fans to use during the day and night.

Wear cool clothing. Use light layers made of natural fibers such as cotton. Avoid nylon, spandex, and some polyesters, which can hold in body heat. Skip satin or all polyester bed sheets.

Use a chill pillow or cold compress. Put something cold around your neck, the inside of your wrists, the inside of your elbows, or between your legs.

Breathe deeply. Try deep, slow breathing (six to eight breaths per minute). Breathe deeply in the morning, evening, and at the onset of hot flashes. According to the North American Menopause Society, deep breathing may be the most effective relaxation method. In three clinical trials, the study reported women who practiced paced breathing had 50 percent fewer hot flashes.[5]

Exercise regularly. Women who are active every day report fewer hot flashes and a shorter duration of hot flashes. Walking, dancing, cycling, and swimming (remember that cool water?) are all good choices.

Smell something soothing. Studies show some scents can calm your body and soothe hot flashes. Calming scents include roses, lavender, vanilla, lemongrass, and essential oils such as geranium and sage.

Avoid triggers such as stress, tight clothing, caffeine, alcohol, spicy foods, heat, and cigarette smoke.

I love what Pam Farrel says about signs that you might be experiencing menopause. Here are two:

- You sell your home heating system at a garage sale.

- Your husband jokes that instead of buying a woodstove, he is using you to heat up the family room this winter.[6]

See, there can be an upside to hot flashes.

Turn Up the Good Stuff

According to Danna Demetre, we all need a healthy lifestyle no matter what. But the woman facing menopause needs it more than ever because her body is going through significant change. Are there foods that can help you navigate menopause more successfully? Thankfully, the answer is yes. During menopause, it's especially important to eat a variety of foods to get the nutrition you need. Follow these dietary guidelines, which are sensible before, during, and after menopause:

Be calcium-rich. An adequate intake of calcium for most women is 1200 milligrams a day. Your body cannot absorb more than 500 milligrams at a time, so spread your calcium intake throughout the day. Eating and drinking two to four servings of dairy products and calcium-rich foods such as broccoli and legumes will help you get enough calcium in your daily diet.

Don't forget the iron. Eat at least three servings of iron-rich foods such as lean red meat, poultry, fish, eggs, leafy greens, or nuts. The recommended dietary allowance for women 19 to 50 is 18 milligrams of iron a day. It's 8 milligrams for women 51 and older.

Fiber up. Enjoy foods high in fiber such as whole-grain breads, cereals, pasta, rice, fresh fruits, and vegetables. Some packaged foods claim to be "rich in fiber" but double-check by reading the label. A good source of fiber should have at least 2.5 grams of fiber per serving. Aim for 20–25 grams of fiber per day.

The war against your hormones can be won. We'll be talking together about good nutrition in the next few days because the fight for your health and sanity is worth it.

Thought for Rejuvenation

What has been your personal experience with menopause?

☐ Not there yet

☐ Sailed through it

☐ Right in the middle of it

☐ Thankful it's behind me

Write a few sentences to describe your experience. If you haven't experienced it yet, what are your expectations?

Act of eXpression

Next time you have an unpleasant symptom such as a hot flash or mood swing, think of a funny memory from your teenage years and be thankful you're not 13 anymore.

Closed for Renovations

Have you ever driven to a store or restaurant only to find a sign on the door, "Closed for Renovations"? Whether it was closed for a minor fix or a major remodel, it was probably an inconvenience to you as a customer. But hopefully you were "wowed" when you saw the finished product a few weeks later.

Do you ever wish you could have a "Closed for Renovations" sign over your life? Wouldn't it be nice to take time out to renovate yourself without any interruptions? If only you could stop the phone from ringing and hit the pause button on your many obligations. Sure it would be inconvenient, but wouldn't it be worthwhile?

Let's just imagine you have a few days without any responsibilities except focusing on the areas in your personal life that need some TLC. What would your renovations list look like?

- Lose 15 pounds
- Get a haircut
- Go through the closet and give away the clothes I haven't worn since 1995
- Plan regular date nights with my husband
- Get my cholesterol under control
- Start walking a few days a week

Permission Granted

Believe it or not, the world will not stop spinning on its axis if you take a short sabbatical. Whether it's a quiet weekend or a six-month period when you don't volunteer for anything, give yourself permission to take care of you. If you're so busy meeting the needs of everyone else and you neglect yourself, who pays when you have a heart attack at age 50 that could have been avoided? You pay and so do the people you've been trying to protect.

Speaker and author Karen Ehman has great advice for setting boundaries:

> What women do when we're presented with an opportunity outside the home is we ask, *Am I capable?* And we think, *Sure, I could do that,* when really we should ask, *Am I called?* When we use capability as our plumb line, we take on way too much. Women have the curse of capability. When someone asks us to put another thing on our plate, we just add it instead of removing something else from our plate to make room.[7]

Does that sound familiar, Miss-multitasker-on-the-verge-of-a-meltdown? If you need a time-out, call a family meeting to talk about your needs. Maybe you could use a day alone to organize your desk so you can see straight. Perhaps you need to talk to your kids about axing an afterschool activity because it's putting too much pressure on the family's schedule. Maybe you need some accountability so you don't just talk about making healthy changes in your life, you actually start making them. Don't just wait for "free time" in your life to make renovations. That free time will never appear unless you create it.

From Size 24 to Size 10

Karen Ehman had to learn some boundary issues the hard way. She was in desperate need of a physical renovation. Although she has written books such as *The Complete Guide to Getting and Staying Organized*, Karen was having trouble managing her weight. As a busy homeschooling mother of three, she didn't take time for exercise and proper nutrition. Instead, like so many women, she relieved her stress through eating. When she tipped the scales at 250 pounds, she knew something had to give.

Two factors led to Karen's major life renovation. First, her health was failing. She had bursitis in her right heel and a torn meniscus in her knee that caused so much pain she had trouble walking across a room. She had high cholesterol, and she struggled with incontinence because of the constant weight on her bladder. She joked that "I squeeze when I sneeze, and I cross when I cough," but underneath the laughter, she wasn't happy. Her husband never nagged her about the weight. But during times alone, he admitted he was afraid of what would happen if she were to die, prematurely leaving him with the three kids.

The second thing that happened was Karen caught a glimpse of herself performing a skit on a DVD for a ministry to moms called Hearts at Home. Karen writes, "I could *not* believe that what I saw on the screen was what people saw every time they looked at me. It was enough to shock me into reality and away from the fridge."

Karen decided to put food in its proper perspective. Food was for nourishment, not for comforting, tranquilizing, or escaping. With a friend, she began at her church a weekly eating and accountability group called Weigh and Pray. In just ten months, she lost over 100 pounds and went from a size 24 to a size 10.[8] Was that a worthwhile, life-changing renovation? You bet. Was it easy? No way.

There are times when you have to totally focus on one area in your personal growth. It could be losing weight, exercising, kicking a smoking habit, praying more intimately, or earning a college degree. Don't simply accept the circumstances in your life that you don't like. Accept the responsibility to *do* something about them—because you're the only one who can.

I Don't Have Anything to Wear

Let's say, like Karen Ehman, you've lost a lot of weight. Now you have a new problem—you don't have anything to wear. This problem is much easier to solve. Maybe it's time for a little shopping spree to update and renovate your wardrobe. I don't have to tell you how many television shows and magazines are dedicated to instructing you on what to wear and what not to wear. So let me just say a few things about renovating your closet.

Your closet changes as you age. In your twenties, you probably didn't have a hefty mortgage and a stack of bills, so you bought trendy clothes instead. You enjoyed following the latest styles and experimenting with different combinations. In your thirties, it became more difficult to have an up-to-date wardrobe at budget prices. In your forties and beyond, you aren't thinking about the hottest fashions anymore. You're thinking strategic dressing—drawing the eye away from your flaws. And why shouldn't you? When you dress to highlight your physical strengths (and hide the other stuff), you appear healthier, younger, and more beautiful.

If you're over forty and you still have the miniskirts you were wearing in your twenties buried somewhere in your closet, it's time to give those away. When weeding out your closet, Karen Ehman suggests sorting into three piles or boxes:

1. *Giveaway*—These are the clothes that don't fit anymore, don't flatter your figure, or don't have anything to match. If you haven't worn an item in two years, it's time to pitch it. You may have emotional ties to the sweater your favorite aunt gave you, but if you don't wear it, toss it (you can take a picture of it first if you're very sentimental).

2. *Throwaway*—These clothes are in such bad shape that even Goodwill won't touch them. This is the pile where you put your underwear with the shot elastic.

3. *Put Away*—These are items that don't belong in your closet. Maybe you have photo albums, trinkets, or projects that need to be moved. Or clothes that belong to a friend that you keep forgetting to return.[9]

Be ruthless in your sorting. When you try on a borderline outfit, ask yourself, *Would I want to run into someone important at the grocery store wearing this?* or *Would it be okay if the paparazzi took my picture in this and plastered it on the cover of a tabloid magazine?* Once you've made some room in your closet, you can purchase a few new pieces that will complement your figure, style, and current wardrobe. It's never too late to renovate your look, so have fun with it.

FASHION DON'TS AFTER FORTY

Don't wear oversized, baggy clothes.

Don't wear low-rise jeans.

Don't wear overalls.

Don't wear your skirts too short.

Don't wear white pantyhose.

Don't wear old-lady prints.

Don't wear overdone details such as gold buttons and gold trim.

Thought for Rejuvenation

Which renovation do you need the most right now?

☐ Health renovation—I need to improve my eating and exercise habits.

☐ Priorities renovation—I need to pare down my current responsibilities and learn how to say no.

☐ Wardrobe renovation—I need a new look.

☐ Other:

Act of eXpression

With that renovation in mind, write down what you will do today, in the next ten days, and in the next ten months to make that renovation a reality.

Today I will:

In the next ten days I will:

In the next ten months I will:

Eat This, Toss That

Like Karen Ehman in yesterday's reading, maybe you need to make some changes in your diet, but you need a friendly push to get started. Your first victory can happen right in the comfort and privacy of your own home, namely in your kitchen. You can do a very simple thing today to dramatically boost your health and drop a few pounds. Are you ready? Throw out the foods and drinks in your kitchen and pantry that stand in the way of optimum health and weight loss. What foods am I talking about? Cookies, chips, milk chocolate, candy bars, cake, soda, sugary drinks, TV dinners, white bread, bagels, and _____ (you fill in the blank).

I said it was simple, not easy.

"The less we eat out of packages, boxes, and cans, the better," says Danna Demetre, RN and author of *Change Your Habits, Change Your Life*. "Try to get back to food as natural as possible. Ramp up on vegetables, fruits and nuts, foods with lots of fiber."[10]

For James and me, our turning point happened when his employer hired a corporate personal trainer, rightly thinking that a healthier employee equaled a more productive employee. James came home with all sorts of new ideas from this personal trainer. We began eating oatmeal instead of bagels for breakfast, fruit instead of sugary snacks, and got rid of the ice cream in the freezer. I wondered what happened to my chocolate-chip-cookie-loving husband, but after a few weeks, I realized how much better I was feeling. My regular headaches were gone. What began as a trial period ended in a new lifestyle we both grew to love.

Shop Smart

Since then, I've been pregnant several times, and junk food has made its way back into our pantry and freezer. The truth is, if you have easy access to something delicious and unhealthy, you will eat it. But if you work—and I mean work—to eliminate junk food from your house, you will reap amazing health benefits. When your refrigerator is stocked with clean, cut fruits and vegetables, you will snack on those things. One battle for your body's health is won in the grocery store. The next time you go grocery shopping, try doing these two things to improve your odds of winning:

1. Do not go shopping when you are hungry. As you know, you'll be more vulnerable to buy whatever looks good, which usually isn't broccoli.

2. Look at the contents of your shopping cart before you check out. Do you picture a fat or skinny person buying these items? Are there more natural foods than packaged foods? Look at each food item and ask yourself, *How will this benefit my body? How will this damage my body? Is it worth the calories?*

If you want to get leaner, you must start by trimming your grocery cart from unnecessary calories, which will make your kitchen and pantry a safer place to eat. Danna Demetre says, "The old cliché 'you are what you eat' is so true. If we are constantly building a new body, from our skin cells that regenerate daily to our blood cells that regenerate monthly to our skeletal system that regenerates completely in seven years, what are you building that all with? What I am tomorrow is what I eat today."[11]

Pantry Patrol

What foods are you using to build your body? If you're like most women, you need to eliminate some of the unhealthy foods available to you at home. (I'm thinking of my secret stash of Thin Mint Girl Scout cookies right now.) If you wanted to purge your pantry of excess salt, sugar, white flour, or bad fats, would you be able to do it? Maybe you're thinking if you lived alone, this might work. But your husband or kids may not appreciate having the pantry patrolled. You may be dubbed "The Health-Food Nazi." Here are a few suggestions for your family:

1. Ask your family to eat healthy with you for a specified length of time. The goal is to rid your home of junk food permanently, but going cold turkey may be a bit much. You can do a trial run first. Try eating healthy at home for one month. It will be hard at first, but by the second week you'll notice a positive difference. Eating healthy will make everyone feel so much better.

2. Put all the junk food in a big box and seal it up with shipping tape. Store it in a closet and don't open it until a certain date or until you lose a certain amount of weight. Label it clearly, "Do not open before May 1" or "Do not open until Mom loses five pounds." By the time you open the box again, you'll hopefully want to give away the food because you have momentum on your side and you're losing weight.

3. If asking your family to give up their junk food is next to impossible, then label the junk food in your house. Put your husband's name on the bag of chips. Your kid's name on the soda can. These things belong to your family; they do not belong to you. They are off limits.

Healthy eating is all about access. It's about eating this and tossing that. My friend Debbie used to have two liters of soda and a bag of chips on hand at all times. After she was diagnosed with breast cancer, she had to completely change her diet. Today, you can't find soda or chips at her house. She's munching on salads these days and cherishing her health.

If you're part of the nearly 30 percent of all women who suffer from adult acne, avoid refined foods such as bread and pasta. Studies have shown these foods increase the production of the hormone androgen, which increases oil production and triggers breakouts. On the other hand, you can improve your skin and ward off wrinkles by eating oranges. Women over 40 who consumed greater amounts of vitamin C were 11 percent less likely to develop wrinkles.[12]

Today is the day to take charge of your physical well-being. If you are what you eat, it's time to choose healthy food and toss out junk food. You're worth it. Smart eating will make you feel great today and for many, many tomorrows to come.

EIGHT SUPER FOODS FOR OPTIMUM HEALTH

Blueberries

Black beans

Spinach

Yogurt

Tomatoes

Carrots

Oats

Walnuts

Thought for Rejuvenation

How would you describe the state of your refrigerator and pantry?

☐ A junk food paradise—whatever you're craving, we've got it.

☐ A vending machine—we have a good selection of junk food to choose from.

☐ A snack pack—we have a few things for when we get the munchies.

☐ A survival kit—just a little junk food for emergencies.

☐ A health-food paradise—junk food is of the devil.

What would it take to purge your pantry? Do you need to ask permission from your husband or kids?

Act of eXpression

Check your current habits against this sample daily eating plan:

Food Group	Examples	Amount
Grains	Oatmeal, bread*	6 oz**
Vegetables	Broccoli, tomatoes	2.5 cups
Fruits	Apples, strawberries	2 cups
Dairy	Yogurt, cheese	3 cups
Meat and Beans	Chicken, turkey, fish	5.5 oz
*One slice of whole-wheat bread is about 35 grams, which is a little more than 1 oz		
**1 ounce = 28.35 grams		

What will you eat today to improve your diet?

1.

2.

3.

What will you skip today to improve your diet?

1.

2.

3.

Day 21

A Fast from Fast Food

After watching the documentary *Super Size Me*, my husband and I never looked at fast food in quite the same way. In the film, director Morgan Spurlock eats nothing but McDonald's for 30 straight days. A five-year-old's dream. He went to McDonald's three times a day, sampled everything on the menu, and "super-sized" his meal whenever the cashier suggested it. The Academy Award-nominated film follows the drastic effect this McDiet had on Spurlock's health and well-being. In just one month of his experiment, he gained 24.5 pounds, experienced terrible mood swings, lethargy, high cholesterol, and signs of liver disease.

Now I understand no one in their right mind goes to McDonald's every day for a month straight. But how many times do you eat fast food per week? How do you measure up against today's average American who eats four or more meals away from home each week? One out of four Americans will eat fast food today, and 43 percent of those people will choose the industry leader, McDonald's.[13]

During the movie, Spurlock showed how the fast-food industry has contributed to a Super-Sized Nation, changing the way Americans eat with large serving sizes and meals of hamburgers, fries, and Cokes. In 1970, Americans spent 6.2 billion dollars at fast-food restaurants. In 2004, that number rose to 124 billion—20 times as much.[14]

Fast food is good business—that's why you're sure to pass several conveniently located fast-food restaurants whenever you drive just about anywhere. Within only five miles of my home in San Diego, there are 13 McDonalds, 10 Subways, 10 KFCs, 7 Burger Kings, and 5 Taco Bells. Talk about convenient.

Depressed at the Drive-Through

My friend Chelle Stafford knows the dangers of hitting the drive-through too often. Her story was featured in the March 2009 issue of *Women's Health* magazine. I hadn't seen her in more than 20 years, so imagine my surprise when I saw her picture in *Women's Health* as a weight-loss success story. After three babies, six miscarriages, and a hysterectomy, she was going through a hard emotional time. Her weight shot up to 178 pounds. Standing in a dressing room trying to find a New Year's Eve outfit, she broke down sobbing. She couldn't get into a size 16, and there was no way she was going up a size. So the day after New Year's, she signed up with a personal trainer.

One of the first orders of business was starting a food journal. Chelle was instructed to write down everything that went into her mouth, and her eyes were opened. "I was eating fast food—McDonald's, Taco Bell, whatever was handy—sometimes three times a day. And this was every day of the week. My salt intake was the biggest shock. I wondered why I hadn't had a heart attack yet."[15]

She decided to slowly ditch the drive-through. Her fast-food visits became less frequent: first once a day, then once a week, and eventually she could flip through her food journal for weeks without seeing fast-food entries.

How did she kick the fast-food habit? She credits her secret weapon—an Igloo Playmate cooler. "I cook healthy meals on Sundays and pack one each weekday, so there's no excuse to hit the drive-through," Chelle said. Her strategy and dedication paid off. In five months, she dropped three sizes.

Remember McDonald's catchy slogan, "You deserve a break today"? Chelle had to learn how to have breaks without French fries and hot-fudge sundaes. Instead, she went on walks, picked up a new book, or went to the gym. By radically improving her diet and exercising five times a week, she reached her goal weight in one year and ten months, dropping a total of 55 pounds. Plus she's free of the inhaler she used to need every day. That's the kind of break she *really* needed.[16]

Is It Really a Happy Meal?

Maybe you're not a fan of fast food, but you have children or grandchildren who are. That's no surprise since corporations spend over 15 billion dollars a year on marketing and promotions to get kids to beg and whine for fast food.[17] From a child's perspective, a fast-food restaurant equals a playground, a cheeseburger, fries, soda, and a toy. To please our kids, and maybe even to feel young ourselves, fast food is a cheap, easy, and fun night out. But with childhood obesity sharply on the rise, buyers beware.

Am I saying that fast food is completely evil and that you and your family should never darken the doors of a fast-food chain? Picking up an occasional burger, taco, pizza, or piece of chicken isn't a problem, but making it a regular habit is. Just look at this list of some of the worst fast foods according to AOL Health (www.aolhealth.com). As you look through these delicious but unhealthy choices, keep in mind the daily recommended allowance of fat is 65 g and sodium is 2400 mg:

- Quiznos Tuna Melt, large: 1760 calories, 133 g fat, 2120 mg sodium

- McDonald's Double Quarter Pounder with Cheese: 740 calories, 42 g fat, 1380 mg sodium

- Taco Bell Grilled Stuft Burrito (beef): 680 calories, 30 g fat, 2120 mg sodium

- Wendy's Bacon and Cheese Baked Potato with all the toppings: 550 calories, 22 g fat, 1080 mg sodium

- Subway Sweet Onion Chicken Teriyaki footlong: 770 calories, 9 g fat, 2290 mg sodium

- Baskin-Robbins Large Chocolate Oreo Shake: 2600 calories, 135 g fat, 263 g sugar, 1700 mg sodium

- Dunkin' Donuts Reduced-Fat Blueberry Muffin: 450 calories, 10 g fat, 670 mg sodium

Oops. I've ordered the Subway Sweet Onion Chicken Teriyaki sandwich without realizing how much salt was in it. Of course there are healthier options at Subway (try the eight-ounce Minestrone Soup and Grilled Chicken and Baby Spinach Salad with Greek vinaigrette). The problem is once you're inside the doors of a fast-food joint, it's easy to cave in and order a bacon cheeseburger with fries and a soda.

If you're meeting friends at a fast-food place or stopping by after church, check out the restaurant's nutritional guide online before going. All the fast-food chains post their menus on their websites with nutritional values listed. Decide what's the best option for you (what sounds appealing and isn't among the worst offenders on the menu) and stick with the plan.

Maybe you eat fast food regularly with coworkers for lunch, or you hit the drive-through more than once a week on your way home for dinner. Now is a good time to consider a fast from fast food. When you replace the sugary, fat-laden, fast-food meal with a healthier alternative, your body will thank you for it.

In Richard Foster's book, *The Celebration of Discipline,* he writes about the discipline of fasting. "Fasting reminds us that we are sustained 'by every word that proceeds from the mouth of God' (Matt. 4:4). Therefore, in experiences of fasting we are not so much abstaining from food as we are feasting on the word of God. Fasting is feasting."[18]

So the next time you crave a value meal at your favorite fast-food place, remember the catchy phrase "fasting is feasting." By skipping unhealthy meals, you will be feasting.

Thought for Rejuvenation

How many times per month do you eat at a fast-food restaurant?

Which fast-food restaurants do you frequent the most?

Act of eXpression

Choose your favorite fast-food place. Go to that company's website and look up the nutritional information for one meal you've ordered before. How many calories? How much fat? Sugar? Sodium?

Do you need to take a fast from fast food? If so, write down your commitment (for example, *In the next month, I will eat fast food only twice*):

Drink and Grow Rich

Every time I fly, I choose a free beverage for two reasons. I don't drink alcohol, and even if I did, I'm too cheap to pay for it. Whenever I see a passenger order a beer or Bloody Mary I think, *Wow, that little drink cost six dollars. That's expensive.* Did you ever think you could grow rich from what you *don't* drink?

James and I (aka Mr. and Mrs. Frugal) always order water at restaurants. James loves to say we're "big drinkers" because we like big glasses of water with our meals. Naturally, this is quite disappointing for our server. One day we calculated how much money we've saved in the past ten years doing this. Assuming we go out an average of twice a month, we have saved $1200. Of course, that's if we had ordered soda, iced tea, or lemonade. If we ordered alcohol, our savings would be even greater. And keep in mind most people eat out a lot more than twice a month. So drinking water isn't just good for your waistline; it's good for your bottom line.

Liquid Health

Think of water as free liquid health. Water gives you energy, helps you lose weight, lowers your risk of heart attack, and improves your skin and teeth—all for free. If you don't get enough of it, you may become dehydrated, which means your body won't have enough water to carry out normal functions. Even mild dehydration can drain your energy and lead to headaches, fatigue, muscle weakness, and dizziness.

Your body is estimated to be about 60 to 70 percent water. Blood is mostly water, plus your brain, muscles, and lungs all contain a lot of water.

Your body needs water to regulate body temperature and transport nutrients to all your organs. Water also brings oxygen to your cells, removes waste, and protects your joints and organs. A six-year study published in the *American Journal of Epidemiology* found that people who drank more than five glasses of water a day were 41 percent less likely to die from a heart attack than those who drank less than two glasses during that study period.[19] You may think you need coffee to start your day, but what you could really use is a glass of water.

Not only does water do wonders on the inside of your body, it helps on the outside too. Drinking plenty of water helps your skin stay elastic and supple. When you're properly hydrated, your skin looks healthier and less wrinkly. So if you want your skin to have a healthy glow, don't forget to reach for eight glasses of water a day. Water also protects your pearly whites because when you drink soda and even sports drinks, they contain acids that erode dental enamel. That's great for your dentist's business, but not so great for you.

Drink Water and Lose Weight

What other drink besides water delivers so many health benefits at zero calories? Water is in a class all by itself. It's one of your best allies for losing weight. Chances are there are times in the day besides mealtimes when you feel hungry. Believe it or not, you may be more thirsty than hungry. By drinking a tall glass of water whenever you feel hungry, you may stop yourself from grabbing that unnecessary snack (or at least reduce the size of that snack). You can also drink a glass of water before your meal to fill your stomach, which will help you to put your fork down sooner.

If you drink a lot of water, you won't be drinking other beverages, such as sugary sodas or high-calorie coffee drinks. Let's say you switch out a caramel frappuccino blended coffee with whipped cream (venti size) with an ice-cold glass of water. You'll save yourself 500 calories—that's about one-fourth of your entire caloric intake for the day—and pass on 68 grams of sugar, which will definitely help your waistline. If you don't want to skip your coffee, try a lower calorie choice such as a small café latte or cappuccino made with fat-free milk (about 120 calories) or have your cup of java black.

Do you like soda? If so, you're not alone; soft drinks are a main staple of the average American diet. Americans spend $80 billion a year on beverages, $64 billion of which is spent on soft drinks. Why is soda not only popular but problematic to your health? Consider that many 12-ounce sodas contain ten teaspoons of sugar. You wouldn't imagine putting ten teaspoons of sugar into your mouth, one spoonful at a time, but it sure is easy to gulp it down with ice.

Studies show that women who drink one or more sodas each day are twice as likely to develop type 2 diabetes in a four-year period as women who drink less than one soda a day. Fructose, which is the sweetener found in many sodas, will make you gain weight, but its replacement isn't much better. Artificial sweeteners such as aspartame have been linked to migraine headaches and other negative health reactions.[20] Danna Demetre, RN, says,

> You think you can't live without your soda, but the truth of the matter is, if you could see on a microscopic level some of the damage, the excessive sugar and chemicals, you would start to think, *I do not enjoy drinking things that are not good for me. And I love drinking things that really nourish my body.* If you tell yourself that little piece of self-talk every day, it will help you have a different attitude about the things you put in your mouth.[21]

But I Don't Like the Taste

You may know the health benefits of water, but when it comes down to it, you just don't like the taste. There are a few things you can add to your glass of water to make it more appealing: lemon or lime wedges, a sprig of mint, strawberries, or even cucumber slices. Sparkling mineral water is also a good alternative, especially if you're weaning yourself off soda. Just make sure the sparkling water you choose has zero calories and no sugar or artificial sweeteners added.

Maybe you're having trouble squeezing eight glasses into a day. Just a few minor adjustments in your daily routine may do the trick:

- Drink a glass of water when you wake up.
- Drink a glass of water with breakfast, lunch, and dinner.
- Carry a water bottle with you when you go out.
- Keep a glass of water on your desk when you're working.
- Have a few extra water bottles in the car.

- Drink a glass of water in the afternoon, between lunch and dinner.

- Drink water before, during, and after exercise.

- Eat foods that naturally contain water, such as watermelons, oranges, grapefruit, and even broccoli and carrots.

If you need more variety in what you drink, here are the next best beverages after water:

Tea (especially green tea). Tea is loaded with antioxidants that help prevent damage to your body. Tea has also been shown to reduce stress and contribute to longevity. You can drink it hot or cold in any season.

Milk (low-fat and fat-free). Milk has calcium and protein, and has been demonstrated to reduce the risk of osteoporosis, hypertension, colon cancer, and kidney stones. Unlike soda, it may also help to reduce the risk of tooth decay instead of contributing to it. Soy milk is a good alternative if you're lactose intolerant.

One hundred percent fruit juice. Make sure there is no sugar added and limit your serving to four to eight ounces. If you're used to drinking much more than that, try diluting the juice with water or adding a little juice to sparkling water for a treat.

Vegetable juice. Vegetable juice is a great low-calorie choice with antioxidants, such as vitamins A and C, and other nutrients such as lycopene. Eight ounces of vegetable juice has two grams of fiber, is very low in sugar, and only 50 calories. Look for low- or reduced-sodium options.

As you choose your drinks wisely and focus on the building block of water, you'll grow rich in health benefits—and your beverage bill won't put a dent in your pocketbook.

Thought for Rejuvenation

Write down your estimate of how many cups you drink per day of the following beverages:

Water _____

Coffee _____

Tea   _____

Milk   _____

Juice   _____

Soda   _____

Other   _____

Act of eXpression

Drink six to eight glasses of water today. If you need a game plan to make that happen, write down your plan here. Feel free to use some suggestions from today's reading.

Day 23

You've Got to Move It

This blog comment caught my eye:

> When I go walking with my mom who is 73, I often have to tell her to slow down so I can catch up. She is also ten times more flexible than I am. When I run, my goal is to beat the senior citizens and the seven-year-olds. Sometimes I succeed.
>
> —Anonymous

Wouldn't it be inspiring to be in your seventies and run faster than your daughter? I thought of my mom when I read that comment. When my mom was in her midfifties, she hadn't exercised in years. She never played sports or watched *Sweatin' to the Oldies* with Richard Simmons. You couldn't pay her enough money to step inside a gym. And then something happened.

My husband noticed that a personal trainer in our neighborhood taught an indoor cycling class in her garage. Indoor cycling is aerobic exercise that takes place on a stationary bike and doesn't require much coordination, which is why my mom was willing to give it a try.

The rigorous class lasts for a brutal 45 minutes, and to my mom's credit, she smiled through the whole thing. Four years later, she's still cycling away twice every week.

"If it wasn't for the indoor cycling class, I would have skipped exercise many weeks," my mom says. "It's become a routine, and I really need that. I think I'd be ten pounds heavier if I didn't go."[22]

I don't think my mom can outrun me, but she might be able to "outspin" me.

How Much Is Enough?

It doesn't matter if you bike, walk, run, or swim. The point is to keep moving. How much physical activity do adults really need? According to the *2008 Physical Activity Guidelines for Americans* published by the U.S. Department of Health and Human Services, adults need at least:

- 2 hours and 30 minutes (150 minutes) of moderate-intensity aerobic activity (i.e., brisk walking) every week

Or

- 1 hour and 15 minutes (75 minutes) of vigorous-intensity aerobic activity (i.e., jogging or running) every week

Plus

- Muscle-strengthening activities on two or more days a week that work all major muscle groups (legs, hips, back, abdomen, chest, shoulders, and arms)[23]

Muscle-strengthening activities can be done at home or in the gym. They include:

- Lifting weights

- Working with resistance bands

- Doing exercises that use your body weight for resistance (push-ups, sit-ups)

- Heavy gardening (digging, shoveling)

- Yoga

If you're thinking, *How can I meet these guidelines each week?* remember you can spread your activity throughout the week. God gives you seven days to get it done. You can even exercise in ten-minute increments and find ways to multitask throughout the day, such as lifting weights while you watch television.

On the other hand, if you're thinking, *No problem; these guidelines are easy,* why don't you challenge yourself to take it to the next level? For even greater health benefits, the *2008 Physical Activity Guidelines for Americans* recommends 5 hours of moderate-intensity aerobic activity or 2 hours and 30 minutes of vigorous-intensity aerobic activity per week. If your workout is intense, you can cut your exercise time in half. Everyone interested in saving time will want to move from moderate activity to vigorous activity.

How do you know if you're doing moderate or vigorous aerobic activity (besides the feeling that you're about to pass out)? Think of a 10-point scale where sitting is 0 and working as hard as you can is 10. Moderate-intensity aerobic activity is about a 5 or 6. You'll be breathing harder and your heart will be beating faster, but you'll still be able to talk. Vigorous-intensity aerobic activity is a 7 or 8 on this scale. You won't be able to say more than a few words without stopping to catch your breath.

Small Steps to Success

Whether you're continuing your exercise regimen or beginning a new one, remember to use common sense. Everyone has different abilities and fitness levels. Do what feels comfortable to you and push yourself accordingly. If you compare yourself to your friend who's winded after one flight of stairs, you might feel like a fitness expert. But when you hear about the friend who just completed a half marathon, you might feel more like a couch potato. Don't compare yourself to others. Instead, compete against yourself, constantly striving to have more endurance, strength, and speed in your personal workouts.

Maybe you'd like to exercise more, but you wonder when you will find the time. Think of it this way. You can pull out your calendar and schedule times for going to the gym, taking a brisk walk, lifting weights at home, or playing sports. Or you can write in extra doctor's appointments and trips to the cardiologist, because that's where you may end up if you don't take care of your body. I think you'll agree that exercise is the more attractive option, so let's start moving today.

Thought for Rejuvenation

How does your exercise routine measure up to the one recommended by the *2008 Physical Activity Guidelines for Americans*?

What types of exercise do you enjoy most?

Act of eXpression

Look at your calendar for the next week. Schedule in 150 minutes of moderate activity or 75 minutes of vigorous activity and two days of strength training.

Goodnight, Baby

Can sleep be considered a hobby? If so, sign me up. Whether it's lying in bed for an extra ten minutes in the morning or taking that beloved Sunday afternoon nap, the supine position with my eyes closed is one of my favorites.

I'm pregnant as I write this book, so sleep is especially prized. I'm an older mom, so the more shut-eye I can fit into the day, the better. But even with my tired body, there are nights I lie awake, a million thoughts running around in my mind.

Chicken thighs are on sale at the grocery store.

Ethan needs to finish his homework tomorrow.

How am I going to write three chapters this week?

I need to write that thank-you note.

Have you ever been there? A woman's mind is forever active. Counting sheep must not be as effective as it once was. According to a National Sleep Foundation survey, more than half of Americans are sometimes unable to fall or stay asleep, and one-third of us experience sleeping problems every night or almost every night. Insomnia is no respecter of persons; it plagues the young and old alike.[24]

I once interviewed a military chaplain named Brad who remembers having insomnia as early as first grade. He had a terrible fear of death because his nanny had a fatal heart attack in his home. Then there were all the Vietnam War images on the television every night. It's no wonder that little boy had trouble sleeping. But when Brad came to know the Lord as an adult, his insomnia disappeared.

Then there was a woman named Michelle who was overwhelmed with an irrational sense of fear as a new mom. Instead of sleeping, she would hover over her sleeping child just to make sure the baby was still breathing. In the middle of night, she would do something that would make most moms cringe. She'd wake up her sleeping baby just to make sure she was all right. A prisoner of worry and anxiety, Michelle didn't know where to turn.

Do you struggle with insomnia some nights or on a regular basis? Some of the factors that may interrupt the ordinary sleep cycle for women include:

- Changes in hormone levels
- Illness
- Medications
- Stress
- Anticipation of something positive or negative
- Lifestyle changes
- Poor sleep environment
- Anxiety
- Depression

Simple Sleep Strategies

Try these simple sleep strategies before reaching for a sleeping pill:

Don't drink caffeine late in the day. Caffeine provides a boost of energy and stimulates your brain—not something you want happening before bedtime.

Don't stare at the clock. If you haven't fallen asleep after about 20 minutes, get out of bed and do something relaxing, such as reading in a different room, until you feel sleepy.

Don't watch the evening news in bed. Set a media curfew in your bedroom for television watching and computer surfing before you retire.

Don't pay your bills in bed. Use your bed for relaxation, not for a desk.

Don't read a murder mystery in bed. You might think the murderer is lurking underneath the covers.

Don't try to conquer the world in 24 hours. Technology has allowed us to work throughout the night, where generations ago, everyone went to sleep when the sun went down. Sacrificing sleep routinely to get more done is a dead end. The trade-off isn't worth it physically and emotionally.

The Power of Routine

Did you know a bedtime routine is just as important for a two-year-old and a fifty-year-old? My kids brush their teeth, put on their pajamas, read a story, share the day's highlights, and end with prayers and "I love you." Your routine might include something warm to drink, relaxing music as you wash your face, reading a Psalm from the Bible, and saying a prayer of thanks to the Lord.

Also, if you go to bed and wake up at the same time every day, it will be much easier for your body to get into a pattern of restful slumber. Make your bedroom as comfortable, dark, and quiet as possible.

De-Stress

Exercise regularly to reduce stress, but don't do any intense exercise before bedtime. However, light stretches are great before bedtime, especially stretching out your calves, which can tense up during the night.

Pay attention to what you do before bedtime. Are the last activities of your day stress relieving or stress producing? If you have something on your mind before you retire, write it down in a journal or to-do list for the next day.

Easy Listening

What happens when you wake up in the middle of the night and can't go back to sleep? Years ago, my husband and I had a secret weapon—an audio cassette of the Bible, read by a baritone voice in "Old King James" style. We used to pop that in the cassette player and be asleep before Genesis chapter 2. It was very soothing. With today's technology, we've graduated to having an iPod on our nightstands. In the middle of the night, I love listening to words of Scripture, which bring peace, rest, and sweet sleep.

Remember Michelle, the mom who couldn't sleep because she was worried about her baby? One night at 2:00 a.m., she turned on the television, and pastor and author David Jeremiah was talking about slaying the giant of worry. "It felt like he was talking to only me," Michelle says. "I figured, who else is watching this at 2:00 a.m.? I know the Lord had sent him." That night, Michelle asked God to help her with her panic attacks. She began to watch Dr. Jeremiah's television program, *Turning Point*, and as she grew spiritually, the worry that plagued her nights began to vanish, and she slept soundly along with her baby.[25]

Why You Need a Good Night's Sleep

There's a myth that adults need less sleep as we get older, but that's just not the case. Women need seven to nine hours of sleep a night, but many women have trouble falling asleep or staying asleep that long. When you're sleep deprived, it's harder to think, concentrate, remember, solve problems, and be pleasant. A chronic lack of sleep also affects our body's endocrine system, which is responsible for regulating appetite. Research shows that a lack of sleep triggers feelings of hunger and that sleeping less than seven hours a night increases one's chances of becoming obese.[26]

In the *Archives of Internal Medicine*, researchers reported that women 45 to 65 who got five or less hours of sleep a night were 50 percent more likely to develop heart disease than women who got eight hours of sleep a night. Studies also show that high blood pressure has been connected with a lack of sleep.[27]

The medical community resoundingly touts the many health benefits of sleep, and why not? Genesis 2:21-22 says, "So the LORD God caused the man to fall into a deep sleep; and while he was sleeping...the LORD God made a woman from the rib he had taken out of the man." That was probably the best thing that ever happened after a good night's sleep, right?

If you ever have trouble sleeping, remember your heavenly Father is waiting "to grant sleep to those he loves" (Psalm 127:2). Goodnight, baby.

Thought for Rejuvenation

Circle the factors that may be hindering your good night's sleep:

Changes in hormone levels

Illness

Medications

Stress

Anticipation of something positive or negative

Lifestyle changes

Poor sleep environment

Anxiety

Depression

Other:

Act of eXpression:

If you have trouble sleeping, what is one idea you will try from today's reading to get a good night's rest?

Day 25

Making Time for Love

W hen Bill Farrel returned to his office after a radio interview about his book, *Let Her Know You Love Her: 100 Ways to Make Your Wife's Day*, he found this phone message: "Hey, I just heard some guy on Mighty Sports 90, and he was talking about some book I need. I think it was something like *100 Ways to Make Your Old Lady's Day*. I think I need that book."[28]

He not only needed the book, he could use a lesson in talking about his spouse. None of us wants to be someone's old lady. But I suppose if we were completely honest, on some days we may feel like an old lady.

To fight against senioritis, begin by "thinking young," as Robin and Jack did in Day 11's reading. What activities made you feel close to your spouse in your younger days? A simple thing like holding hands again can do wonders. When James and I were first dating, we held hands everywhere we went. The warmth of his hand pressing against mine thrilled me and made me feel tingly all over. After having kids, I think I held my kid's hands more often crossing the street or walking through a parking lot. But when I remembered to reach out for the hand of my spouse, the warmth of those first days returned.

I'm Not in the Mood

When life goes into overdrive, sex tends to take a backseat. Many women are just plain exhausted from working, caring for children, volunteering, planning grown children's weddings, or scraping up enough money for college tuition. Add menopause to the mix and it can complicate things even further.

When you stop ovulating, you forfeit that regularly scheduled boost in your sex drive. You lose estrogen, which had been working in your favor to elevate mood and interest in sex. Estrogen also works to increase sensation, making sex more pleasurable. Over time, vaginal tissue begins to dry and shrink, making intercourse more uncomfortable. "This can be easily remedied by use of an artificial lubricant," writes Ed Wheat, MD, in his book *Intended for Pleasure*. "You can avoid the problem by taking estrogen or using a vaginal cream containing estrogen, which is absorbed through the vaginal wall."[29]

In addition to the physical changes happening on the inside of your body, changes are happening on the outside too. Graying hair, wrinkles, and a few extra pounds can make you feel less attractive to your spouse. Pam Farrel, coauthor of *Red-Hot Monogamy*, suggests scheduling a little bit of quiet time, taking a 20-minute nap, soaking in a bubble bath, or changing into your favorite outfit that makes you feel sexy to get in the mood. "Your marriage needs you to invest in it, so it's richer and hotter in life's second half. If you take a little extra time and TLC for yourself to accomplish this, it's a worthy spiritual goal," says Farrel.[30]

He's Not in the Mood

Maybe it's not your libido that's shutting down but your husband's. He used to want to make love all the time, but now he's more interested in the nightly news. You may feel rejected or puzzled by your husband's lack of interest, but don't focus on yourself. Instead, try to understand what's going on with your husband and help him in a loving, unselfish, undemanding manner. Dr. Wheat sheds light on the subject for men over 50:

> The man over fifty must accept normal changes in his sexual capabilities. If he tries to hold himself to his twenty-one-year-old performance, he will at times fail and may experience acute anxiety. If he adapts gracefully to minor physiological changes, he can enjoy sex for many years to come. He should remember that what he has "lost" in youthful vigor, he has gained in capacity to express his love in a mature, more meaningful, and more skillful manner.[31]

You are the most important person when it comes to making your husband feel completely capable and comfortable with lovemaking. So what can you do to enjoy more intimacy with your spouse?

Intimacy Stokers

Talk About It. Some good friends (who will remain unnamed) asked us a funny question the first time we had dinner together. They said, "So, where is the craziest place you ever did it?" My husband and I are pretty open, but we had never answered a question like that before at a restaurant. Needless to say, there was lots of laughter, *partial* disclosure, and a close friendship was born.

It may be a bit inappropriate to talk about your sex life with friends, but it should be a comfortable subject of conversation with your spouse. "One of the most erotic things you can do is talk about what you want in bed," Pam Farrel says. Here are a few questions she suggests:

- What do you enjoy?
- What have been your most memorable moments in the bedroom this year?
- Why did that mean so much to you?[32]

The more you think and talk about intimacy, the more you have intimacy. You get more of what you measure.

Be Creative. My friend Lori is a busy homeschooling mom with six children (some grown, some still at home), yet she and her husband, Don, have been able to keep a steady date night for the past 24 years. Once a week after dinner, the kids would have a special movie night while Lori and Don had a romantic date at home (or out when the kids were older). They would eat together over candlelight, talk, and enjoy each other's company. It didn't take much money, but it has paid tremendous dividends. I can attest to the newlywed like quality of their love and affection for each other.

When it comes to physical intimacy, make it a priority to spend quality time together, no matter how busy you are. Be willing to try different things. If you feel stuck in a rut with your lovemaking, try changing the location, mood music, or what you wear. Use massage oil or an aromatic candle, anything to provide a unique experience. I once tried to do a "Dance of the Seven Veils," but it was more of a comedy act than a sexy show. First, I don't know how to belly dance, and second, I didn't have any veils. I used handkerchiefs, bandanas, sarongs, and even a winter scarf. It wasn't sexy, but it was funny.

Use Anticipation. Send your spouse a love note to let him know Friday night is going to be a special night. You can send him a manila envelope with sexy underwear in it. Or send him five notes over five days, complimenting him each day about something you appreciate. When you put sex on the calendar and set it up as a main event, it gives you and your spouse something fun to look forward to.

Don't let this joke depict your sex life after midlife:

> An older couple was lying in bed one night. The husband was falling asleep, but the wife was in a romantic mood and wanted to talk.
>
> She said, "You used to hold my hand when we were courting."
>
> Wearily he reached across, held her hand for a second and tried to get back to sleep.
>
> A few moments later she said, "Then you used to kiss me."
>
> Mildly irritated, he reached across, gave her a peck on the cheek and settled down to sleep.
>
> Thirty seconds later she said, "Then you used to bite my neck."
>
> Angrily, he threw back the bed clothes and got out of bed.
>
> "Where are you going?" she asked.
>
> "To get my teeth."[33]

Thought for Rejuvenation

There's a huge difference between being tolerated and being wanted. Do you tolerate or want your husband sexually? Does it feel like he tolerates or wants you?

Act of eXpression

Talk about this chapter with your spouse. Use some of Pam Farrel's suggested questions:

What do you enjoy?

What have been your most memorable moments in the bedroom this year?

Why did that mean so much to you?

Plan a date night that includes unhurried, intimate time with your spouse.

Am I Too Old to Sparkle?

When Kathy Martin was 30, she experienced a turning point that changed her life. She decided to go for a jog with her husband who, unlike Kathy, was a regular runner. It wasn't long before she literally lay down in the middle of the road exhausted. She remembers her husband saying, "Get up, a car's going to hit you!" to which she joked back, "I hope it does."

She didn't get hit by a car that evening, but she did get bit by a bug—a running bug. It was a real aha moment in her life. She thought, *If I can't run a mile and I'm only 30 years old, I won't be able to walk by the time I'm 60.* With her competitive nature awakened, the next day she ran again, pushing herself to one more telephone pole or one more mailbox. The first 30 days, she didn't enjoy running, but she knew it was something she had to do. Her carrot when running? She would dream of having ice cream afterward.

Kathy's covered a lot of ground since then, and you can't tell from looking at her that she loves ice cream. Today at 58 years old, Kathy has competed in more than 900 races, setting new records in her age group and winning a number of prestigious running awards. In 2002, she ran the mile in 5 minutes, 22.74 seconds at the USA Track and Field National Masters Indoor Championships, a world-record time for women age 50-54. She was selected as the BENGAY Masters Athlete of the Year in 2004, the year she broke seven American records and three world records in the women's 50-54 age group. Not bad for a woman who barely could run a mile at the beginning of her running career.[34]

Just Do It

I had the honor of meeting Kathy at a Mastermind Summit conference in San Diego. My husband said to me, "There's Kathy Martin. She's on that Nike ad and she's in her fifties." I couldn't believe the young, thin, energetic woman he was pointing to was in her fifties. She was living, breathing proof that you're never too old to sparkle.

Her age-defying athleticism caught Nike's attention. Nike asked her several times to be in a television commercial before she reluctantly agreed. In the Nike advertisement, the camera follows Kathy from behind as she's running through the woods, focusing on her fit body in slow motion. You hear Kathy's voice: "See that? It's 51 years old—51 years old and it can run a 5:08 mile. Can I do a 5:02?" The ad ends by revealing Kathy's face, slightly wrinkled with a few gray hairs around the temples.

You don't have to be in your thirties to be in the best shape of your life. Kathy Martin, now 58, is living proof that you can sparkle at any age.

Are You Diaphanous?

I'm not enough of a wordsmith to know what *diaphanous* means. My best guess would have been one of my son's dinosaurs. But nothing could be further from the truth. According to Merriam-Webster, *diaphanous* means "characterized by such fineness of texture as to permit seeing through, characterized by extreme delicacy of form."

I was introduced to *diaphanous* because it was Patsy Clairmont's "Word of the Month" on her website:

> You see *diaphanous* means light, delicate, translucent...like Cinderella's ball gown. Remember how its delicate layers gently rustled as she waltzed with the prince and how it sparkled flecks of light? I sometimes imagine that angels are diaphanous. Don't you? With gossamer wings and a shimmering glow. Really shouldn't we be? This is a brutal, dark, hard world, and we are called to be its dichotomy: light-bearing, delicate in our treatment of others, and translucent in the sense of honesty and vulnerability.[35]

If you've ever seen Patsy speak, then you know she is diaphanous. She sparkles with incredible imagination, energy, love, and zest for life. I remember going to my first Women of Faith conference and hearing Patsy tell the story of buying something at a department store. The young lady at the cash-register sized Patsy up as an average grandmother and began speaking loudly and slowly, "If you have your grandchild, go onto the Internet; you can fill out a survey and get a coupon." Patsy quickly retorted, "I can do that myself. I have my own email and website, thank you. I blog, Facebook, and even Twitter."[36] You go, Patsy!

What Not to Wear

Now there are some sparkly things you should avoid if you're not 20 anymore. Looking younger doesn't mean accessorizing so heavily that you look like an overdone Christmas tree. Just a little bling goes a long way, so skip the sparkly earrings *and* the sparkly necklace *and* the sparkly rings *and* the sparkly bracelet. Pick just one sparkly item to wear at a time if you're going to sparkle. Here are a few other things 20-year-olds can get away with but you shouldn't try as you age:

- Avoid bright or dark lipstick
- Avoid drawing attention to your eyelids with frosted shadow
- Avoid bright nail polish or lots of big rings if your hands are showing signs of aging
- Avoid exposing too much skin
- Avoid heavy perfume
- Avoid oversized earrings
- Avoid jeans with jeweled embellishments

On the flip side, you don't want to age yourself either. Avoid looks that say, "I'm getting old." Say goodbye to:

- Overly matchy outfits (jacket and pants with the same floral print)
- Fake nails
- Holiday sweaters with bells, reindeers, teddy bears, pumpkins, etc.
- Souvenir T-shirts and baggy sweats

- Shoulder pads
- Muumuus
- Elastic waist pants
- Oversized turtlenecks

My stylish 65-year-old friend Jane went into the shoe department at Nordstrom. She observed that many women were no longer wearing flesh-colored pantyhose, so she asked the salesperson about it. The young lady answered, "It's true that young women are no longer wearing nude panty-hose, but women your age are still wearing them." That was the last time my spunky friend wore pantyhose.[37]

Whether you're forty, sixty, or eighty, you can still glow with radiance and confidence. When you approach life with passion and grace, you open up a world of new adventures and possibilities.

SPARKLE, DON'T SLUMP

Do you have the bad habit of slumping? When you stand up straight, you can seemingly lose five pounds instantly. So keep your head up, hold your shoulders up and back, and walk briskly. You'll look and feel more confident with very little effort.

Thought for Rejuvenation

Could someone describe you as *diaphanous* (light-bearing, delicate in your treatment of others, and translucent in the sense of honesty and vulnerability)?

Act of eXpression

Is there something you've put off doing because you believe you're too old? What is it, and what is standing in the way?

Are you using age as an excuse? Is there a valid medical reason holding you back?

Remember Kathy Martin's perseverance in running. What is one thing you will do this week to begin a new adventure?

The Eyes Have It

When was the last time you looked in the mirror only to see tired, puffy, droopy eyes in the reflection? If the eye is the window of the soul, sometimes the windows need to be polished. Instead of *sparkling* with life, your eyes communicate *survival*. And there's good reason for it. You are just plain worn-out with heavy demands on your time and energy.

In their book *Captivating*, John and Stasi Eldredge diagnose part of the problem as too many responsibilities:

> [The church's] message to women has been primarily "you are here to serve. That's why God created you: to serve. In the nursery, in the kitchen, on the various committees, in your home, in your community." Seriously now—picture the women we hold up as models of femininity in the church. They are sweet, they are helpful, their hair is coiffed; they are busy, they are disciplined, they are composed, and they are *tired*.[38]

Can you relate? Of course, meaningful service is an important component of living for God and looking younger, but *too much service* can lead to exhaustion. Many of us aren't very good at setting boundaries (that would be you if you've thought recently, *Why did I say yes to that?*). When you're tired, it's impossible to have young eyes that sparkle with beauty, wonder, and kindness. No amount of makeup can transform sleepy, tired eyes—although the right eye makeup certainly doesn't hurt.

The Quick Fix

To brighten your eyes, keep the eyeliner on your upper lids a little more intense than the liner on your lower lids. When your lower lids have a thick line of eyeliner, it can weigh your eyes down and make you look even more tired. Don't use a heavy hand when putting on eyeliner.

When you apply eye shadow, use a light shade from the top of your upper lid to underneath your eyebrow. Use a medium shade on your eyelid, extending just above the crease. Then apply the darkest shade of eye shadow from the center of your eyelid to the outer corners. The most important step is to blend, blend, blend. Nothing will date you like harsh eye shadow that's not blended in.

To diminish dark circles and puffiness around your eyes, try:

Two Cucumber Slices: Lie down for ten minutes with a slice of cucumber over each of your closed eyes. The coolness of the cucumber soothes tired eyes and provides moisture. It's a great way to relax and refresh your eyes after a day looking at the computer or before a party. If you don't have cucumbers on hand, you can do the same thing with a washcloth soaked in cold water. Wring out the cold washcloth and put that over your eyes for the same cooling effect, which reduces puffiness.

Ice 'Em: To instantly wake up your eyes (and the rest of you too), put an ice cube on your eyelids and under your eyes.

Eye Cream: The skin around your eyes absorbs the water in regular moisturizer, causing more puffiness. Eye creams hydrate without swelling.

Get Your Zs: The best thing you can do to cure dark circles and puffiness is to sleep eight hours a night.

The Eternal Fix

There's something infinitely more essential to beautiful eyes than applying makeup and reducing puffiness. It's found in the words of Jesus in Luke 11:34-35: "Your eye is the lamp of your body. When your eyes are good, your whole body also is full of light. But when they are bad, your body also is full of darkness."

What does it mean that your eye is the lamp of your body? Your eyes enable you to make use of light, allowing you to see where you are and where you want to go. But when something is wrong with your eyes, your body can't make use of even the most radiant light. I remember when a teenager at my church got poked accidentally in the eye with a coat hanger; he had to stay home to rest that eye. He couldn't see to do his homework, practice the piano or drums, or get something to eat.

Similar limitations happen when your spiritual eyes are injured. You cannot see where to put your feet to walk or how to perform your work. Maybe you have a critical spirit about everything and everyone. Perhaps you can relate to the person who sees the speck in his brother's eye without noticing the plank in his own eye (Matthew 7:2-4). When your inward attitude is wrong toward others, God, and yourself, you shut out the light of Christ in your life.

On the flip side, when your desires, intellect, and actions are controlled by the Holy Spirit, you will experience spiritual illumination. You'll be like the person with perfect eyesight who can see clearly where to go and what to do. When your eyes are spiritually healthy, you will:

- Be blessed and bountiful (Proverbs 22:9)
- Fix your eyes on the eternal, not the temporary (2 Corinthians 4:17-18)
- Know the hope, riches, and great power for those who believe (Ephesians 1:18-19)
- Look forward to when God will wipe every tear away (Revelation 21:4)

When you walk closely with Christ, your eyes will be bright and youthful, sending out a warm invitation to everyone who crosses your path. Glamour icon Sophia Loren said, "Beauty is how you feel inside, and it reflects in your eyes. It is not something physical."[39] I would add, "It's something spiritual."

What Do You See?

My music pastor Joel Marple was one of five children raised by a single mom, and he was part of a school lunch program. Every day, the kids who could pay for their lunches got a white ticket, and the kids who were being subsidized by the school got a brown ticket. He was so ashamed of that brown ticket and always hid it in his pocket until the last minute. He didn't want to be known as the welfare kid.

One day, a woman on staff walked up to him and handed him a roll of shiny white tickets. "Here, I bought these for you. Go stand in the other line and enjoy your lunch." To this day, he remembers the kindness of that woman and the day he got to use the white tickets.

Do you have eyes to see the needs of the people around you as that woman did?

In his book, *Windows of the Soul,* Ken Gire describes how Jesus was able to see beyond what others saw.

> Beyond the widow's tears for her dead son, Jesus saw how much she needed that son to fill the hole left by her deceased husband. Beyond the Samaritan woman's veil, He saw the five marriages that had failed, and beyond that, the emptiness in her life that grew bigger with each divorce. Beyond the power and wealth of Zacchaeus, He saw a small man with a big hole in his heart that all the power and wealth in the world couldn't fill.[40]

When you see others with the love and care of Christ, your eyes will sparkle at any age.

BEAUTY TIP: UPDATE YOUR EYEWEAR

Drop the dated frames, frames that droop downward, and the eyeglass necklace. Glasses can make or break your look because of their prominence on your face. Shop for a new pair of hip, attractive frames every few years (it's not only fashionable, but you need to check your prescription anyway). My friend Kay likes to get ideas in magazines for frames that look good, and then she chooses the most stylish, young person at the optometrist's office to assist her in selecting frames.

Thought for Rejuvenation

To add youth and vitality to your eyes, do you need more of a quick fix or an eternal fix? Why?

Act of eXpression

Read the story in Matthew 20:29-34 of Jesus healing two blind men. Do you need Jesus to touch your eyes today? Pray that He will revive your eyes and give you the spiritual insight you need.

The Best Thing You Can Wear

Recently I was in an elevator at a department store with my two young children. A young 20-something male employee stood sullenly inside the elevator. With a big smile on my face, I prompted my oldest to ask him how his day was going. Without looking up, the employee mumbled, "This is my second job today." I empathized, and then said brightly, "At least you have work." The elevator doors opened and he shuffled out lazily, never making eye contact or smiling at us once.

The encounter actually made me giggle as I whispered to my son, "Boy, he was very grumpy." I wanted to take advantage of that teachable moment because I don't want my children to grow up to be sulky 20-year-old employees. The most important thing my kids can wear isn't bought with money—it's a smile.

Most likely you've seen a well-dressed, stylish, fit older woman wearing a very sour expression. A smile makes all the difference in the world, doesn't it? It's the cheapest and easiest way to improve your looks instantly. A smile is contagious, crossing all races and languages. It has the power to transform the plainest woman into a noticeable beauty.

Mother Teresa said, "Every time you smile at someone, it is an action of love, a gift to that person, a beautiful thing."[41] An unknown author said, "A smile confuses an approaching frown." That's truly been the case with author and speaker Thelma Wells. Life gave her many reasons to frown, yet she has learned how to turn that frown upside down.[42]

The Story of Mama T's Smile

There wasn't even a proper name on her birth certificate. Baby Girl Morris was born to an unwed teenage mother who was kicked out of her house. Later this baby was named Thelma and often left with her grandmother, who would lock little Thelma in a dark, smelly, insect-infected closet for hours. Thankfully, Thelma had other relatives—great-grandparents— who loved her and taught her about Jesus. At the age of four, Thelma accepted Jesus and learned how to sing praises to God when locked in that dark closet.

"I would get out of the closet and I had no trauma, no confusion, no bitterness," Thelma said. "God met me as a little girl at the point of my need and covered me with protection. When I got out of the closet, I was able to smile."

Because of God's deep joy in her heart, Thelma Wells grew up to beat the odds, becoming the first black woman to become an assistant vice president of a commercial bank, a popular Women of Faith conference speaker for 12 years, and author of numerous books, such as *Don't Give In... God Wants You to Win.* Today, Thelma is 68 and not slowing down. She's launched her own Ready to Win conferences where she shows women how to live in victory as children of God. She's affectionately called "Mama T."

Baby, I Love to Smile.

Mama T loves to say, "Baby, I love to smile." When you smile, you release feel-good, painkilling endorphins and serotonin in your body. A smile has been proven to lower your blood pressure, boost your immune system, and lower stress levels. No wonder it says in Proverbs 17:22 that "a cheerful heart is good medicine."

Smiling makes you attractive and more youthful. My mom loves to smile, so it's no surprise that people enjoy her company. You want to be near people who smile because joy is contagious and life-giving. If you're a wife and/or mother, you have a responsibility to create an atmosphere of joy in the home. Thelma Wells says, "You cannot create an atmosphere of joy if you are frowning, fussing, screaming, yelling, putting people down, and being a perfectionist."

Your Reason to Smile

Maybe you've had a rough life or you're going through a hard time right now (those crazy hot flashes) and you find it difficult to smile. When Thelma was diagnosed with cancer a few years ago, she didn't feel like smiling very much. "I started griping, whining, and behaving like a victim," Thelma admitted. After a season of being miserable, God spoke to her in her spirit.

"He told me to stop being stupid. Preach to yourself and live what you preach. He asked me, 'Do you know who you are? Do you know who I am? I am the God who suffered, bled, and died for you. I got up from the grave with the keys to your situation in My hand. Take these keys and walk through the door.'"

After the Lord spoke to her, Thelma found her smile and her song once again. She says that smiling isn't a result of everything going right. She's experienced her share of disappointments and brokenness. She's been wrongfully accused, betrayed by friends, and overwhelmed by grief. But she says, "Because we are fearfully and reverently made, according to Psalm 139:13-17, God has placed in each one of us the ability to smile."

Your Anti-Aging Weapon

Smiling is your most powerful weapon in your anti-aging arsenal. You can be thin and grumpy and you'll still look old. But a genuine smile covers a multitude of flaws and makes you look young. Plus smiling is a great way to keep wrinkles away. At 68 years old, Thelma Wells doesn't have wrinkles, not because of a fancy anti-aging skin serum but because of that trademark smile.

The next time you're in front of a mirror, try this experiment. Frown and notice what it does to your face. See the wrinkles on your forehead, under your eyes, and around your mouth. Then smile and feel how your face instantly relaxes and unwrinkles itself. It takes your muscles more work to frown than to smile, so take the easy road and smile.

Fake It to Make It

Earlier I shared a story about teaching my two-year-old daughter to smile. Even when she's not in a happy mood, I can say, "Show me your smile," and she'll fake a little smile. Sure it's not sincere, but it is a start. Usually within a few minutes, her whiny voice is gone and she's back to her cheerful self. Like my daughter Noelle, you can fake a smile too, and before long, it will be the genuine article. By forcing a smile, you can trick your body into believing all is well, reducing stress and tension. It's like flipping a switch; smiling can actually elevate your mood.

Let's see those pearly whites. Why don't you try a smile right now?

BEAUTY TIP

To brighten teeth, use a teaspoon of baking soda with one or two drops of hydrogen peroxide. Brush it on and let it sit for a few minutes, and then rinse. Be sure not to swallow the paste. Also, remember to floss daily, have regular dental check-ups, and use good brushing habits, which will brighten your smile. Don't smoke or drink too much coffee or tea to prevent staining your teeth.

Thought for Rejuvenation

Complete this sentence: I can smile because…

Act of eXpression

Be conscious of your facial expressions today. Do you smile when you see others? Do you smile when you're home alone? Make a conscious effort to smile often today, even if you don't feel like it.

Saving Your Skin

My friend Shari has a funny story about meeting her husband, Tim. They were both pastors' kids, and at one convention, their fathers exchanged pictures and phone numbers of their grown children. Shari was an elementary school teacher in Texas, and Tim a physician in Southern California. They enjoyed talking on the phone, so a face-to-face meeting was arranged. Shari would fly to sunny California to pay a visit.

Shari looked at her pale skin with concern and decided she should go to a tanning booth before meeting Tim. With great enthusiasm, she went every day for two weeks, and now kissed by a bronze complexion, she was ready to meet her dream doc. Imagine her surprise when she saw Tim waiting for her at the airport. He was even paler than she had been.

Tim avoids the sun like the plague, and his first thought was, *Oh no, she's a sun worshipper. This isn't going to work.* Thankfully, the story ends on a happy note of holy matrimony, and Shari hasn't visited a tanning booth since.

Did you ever go to tanning booths in your younger days? Bronze bodies are the rage of youth, but then there's a price to pay in the golden years. Dermatologist Doris J. Day, author of *Forget the Facelift*, says, "Tanning used to be considered a sign of good health. It is now known to be quite the opposite for your skin...To get a tan, the skin must be damaged. There is no such thing as a healthy tan."[43] Whether you get that nice golden look from the sun or the tanning booth, it's not good for your skin.

Does that mean you should become a hermit and just dash from one indoor location to the next? No, you still want to enjoy outdoor activities such as walking, golf, tennis, and picnics with friends. The idea is to take reasonable precautions to protect your skin by avoiding the following dangers.

Danger 1: Sun

Excessive sunbathing and overexposure to the sun damages your skin, increases your risk of skin cancer, and results in freckling and wrinkling. So before you go outside, use this checklist to save your skin:

- Use a sunscreen with an SPF of 30 or higher on your face and body.

- Avoid the sun between 10:00 a.m. and 4:00 p.m. when possible.

- Wear a hat to protect your face.

Danger 2: Smoke

Smoking isn't bad for just your lungs; it's bad for your skin too. Nicotine causes blood vessels to constrict, preventing oxygen and nutrients from getting to your skin. Smokers often look pale and unhealthy as a result. Wrinkles, fine lines around the mouth, and stained teeth and fingers make smokers look much older than they really are. If you need extra motivation to kick the habit, try vanity. You don't want crow's feet, sunken cheeks, and a grayish complexion holding you back.

Danger 3: Salt

Did you know that salt can result in puffy bags under your eyes? When you have too much salt in your diet, you retain water, resulting in those troublesome puffy bags. To decrease your salt intake, start by taking the saltshaker off your kitchen table. Limit your trips to the drive-through since fast food is laden with salt. Read the labels on your foods and you might be surprised at how much salt is in your crackers, cereals, bread, and canned soups and vegetables.

On average, Americans consume about 6000 mg or one teaspoon of salt per day. Guidelines suggest the limit for the average person should be 3000 mg or half a teaspoon or less.[44] Instead of reaching for the saltshaker, reach for a glass of delicious water. Your skin will stay firm and glowing as you stay properly hydrated. You can even spritz your face lightly throughout the day with a spray bottle of water.

Skin-Saver Suggestions

Walking through the facial cleanser aisle at a drugstore or the cosmetics counter at a department store can be overwhelming. Which products should you buy to wash, exfoliate, scrub, moisturize, and protect your skin? How many products does one really need to get a clean face? I like the motto "keep it simple" even when it comes to your skin regimen. If you make skincare too complicated, you probably won't regularly use all of your products.

In the morning: Use a gentle cleanser to wash your face. Use a circular motion and rinse or wipe off with a washcloth and warm water. Follow with moisturizer with an SPF of at least 15. If you want extra protection from the sun, add a layer of sunscreen.

In the nighttime: Use the cleanser and moisturizer again. You don't have to put lotion on your nose if it's already oily. Try to wash and moisturize your face 30 minutes before you go to bed so your moisturizer will sink into your face and not your pillow.

Once a week: Use an exfoliating scrub on your face.

Once a month: Use a firming mask. You can even make one yourself with ingredients you have around the house:

Yogurt Face Mask

Ingredients:

1 tablespoon natural yogurt at room temperature
   (not low-fat or nonfat)

1 teaspoon honey (if needed, microwave for a
   few seconds to soften)

What to do:

Combine ingredients, then apply to face.

Let it sit for 15 minutes.

Wash face with steaming washcloth.

My Italian Mother-in-Law's Secret

My mother-in-law, Marilyn, has beautiful skin. Her friends have asked how she has kept such a nice complexion, and she's been gracious enough to allow me to share her recipe with you. Two simple words: olive oil. She learned about the beauty of olive oil from her friend Dina, who learned it from her Italian grandmother. She uses a little olive oil (the regular kind, not extra virgin) on her face every morning and night, washing it off with cold water. She puts the olive oil in a pump, just as you would do with hand soap. Then she uses a little bit each day and night to wash off her makeup. She's been doing it for more than 20 years now. And you thought olive oil was good only for cooking.

While we're on the subject of cooking, let me close with one last tip to save the skin on your hands. When you wash the dishes or use household cleaners, wear a pair of gloves. As you age, your hands produce less oil and lose their ability to hold onto moisture, so save your skin and put on some gloves.

Thought for Rejuvenation

Which danger poses the biggest personal threat to the health of your skin: sun, smoke, or salt? What's one thing you could change in your life to preserve your skin?

Act of eXpression

Use a facial mask (you can try the yogurt mask from today's reading) and enjoy a few minutes of relaxation today.

Spa Day

I must admit I haven't been much of a spa girl. My idea of pampering is putting clear nail polish on my fingernails. I have been to a spa only once in my life when I was given a gift certificate to a posh local spa and resort.

I walked through the landscaped courtyard into a new tranquil world of brown sugar and Dead Sea salt scrubs, Egyptian milk baths and Lily body wraps. I began by sitting in the Jacuzzi, since I knew how to do that. Then I went for a face, neck, and shoulder massage. Modest by nature, I kept my underwear on beneath the white towel cover-up given to me.

After the massage, I was led into a steamy room and instructed to lie facedown on a table. The floor was wet, and I was a little nervous about what would happen next. With the cover-up still over my body, a woman began massaging me with a jet spray of water. Think human car wash. I was mortified, not because of the hydra-massage, but because I was still wearing my underwear. It would be only a matter of time before Victoria's Secret would not be a secret anymore. I was so embarrassed when the woman peeled off my wet towel to replace it with a warm and dry one, only to find me wearing soaked underwear. Of course, she was well-trained and didn't even smirk.

Back in the dressing room, I didn't know what to do. The underwear was worth keeping, but how would I leave the elegant spa holding a pair of wet undies? I didn't have a bag with me or a purse large enough to put them in. So I decided to wring them out and wear them under my jeans. I remember driving home in wet underwear thinking, *This was hardly relaxing.* I felt as though I were on an episode of *I Love Lucy*. Next time, I'll know better to wear only the white terry towel.

Spa Sensation

Like me, you may be unfamiliar with the spa world, or you may be like millions of Americans who feel at home with body wraps, facials, and massages. According to a survey by the American Massage Therapy Association, 21 percent of adult Americans receive at least one massage each year.[45] The International Spa Association reports that one-quarter of all American adults have had at least one visit to a day spa, weekend spa, or week-long spa getaway.[46] Who wouldn't want to look like the beautiful, relaxed people always featured in spa advertisements? Many spa treatments can reduce stress, relieve pain, and simply help you feel rejuvenated. It's not surprising that most spa treatments involve human touch, which is a key element in helping people relax and feel better.

But the spa world isn't completely sunny. Bacteria love hot, wet environments, which means bacteria can thrive in those relaxing heated pools, warm baths, and sauna rooms. Manicures and pedicures can also be risky if the instruments are not properly cleaned. For that reason, if you receive a manicure or pedicure, you may want to bring your own instruments if you have them.

Pampering also comes with a price tag, anywhere from a 30-minute back and neck massage for $55 to a 3-hour spa package for $450. Or:

- Swedish body massage: $80/hour

- Deep-tissue massage: $100/hour

- Seaweed body wrap: $90/hour

- Deep-cleansing facial: $80/hour

WHEN YOU VISIT THE SPA

Don't be afraid to ask questions or ask how to get around the spa facility.

Communicate your preferences for room temperature and in-room music selection, and tell your therapist of any skin irritations.

Drink plenty of water after any massages.

Avoid showering directly after a treatment so your body can absorb any oils or lotions.

Spa for Cents

If you don't want to spend so much money for the spa experience, you can create your own spa at home. Granted it would be quite a feat to turn your home into the spa at the Four Seasons, but with a little bit of fuss, you can transform a room of your home into a relaxing getaway.

Begin by choosing your spa location—maybe your bedroom and bathroom or the living room and kitchen area. De-clutter the area since it's hard to relax while staring at a pile of laundry or stack of bills. Wait for a time when you have the house all to yourself. If there is no such time, then ask your husband or other family members to go out for a few hours one night.

Set the mood with music. Most day spas have relaxing sounds piped in of ocean waves, falling rain, or nature. You can purchase a nature-sounds CD or listen to anything you find calming. I like instrumental worship, acoustic guitar, piano, or classical music. Change the lighting in the room by using candlelight. Purchase a big, fluffy towel that you use just for spa day.

Here are a few ideas to get you started with your home spa:

Sweet Sugar Scrub

Ingredients:

¼ cup granulated sugar

2 tablespoons light oil, such as almond, canola, or sunflower

2 tablespoons milk

Mix together all the ingredients into a smooth cream. Before bathing, massage the mixture all over your body to remove dry, flaky skin and increase circulation. Make sure you are in the bathtub, shower, or standing on a towel. Rinse your skin with warm water, then moisturize and enjoy.

Fabulous Footbath

Ingredients:

1 tablespoon sea salt

1 tablespoon honey

5 drops of lavender oil or peppermint oil

Pour the sea salt into a small bowl. Add honey and gently stir the mixture. Drop in the oil and continue to stir. Fill a footbath with comfortably hot water. You can use a plastic bin or even a roasting pan for your footbath. Scoop the mixture into the footbath. Use your feet to move it around. Relax and soak your feet for about 30 minutes. Dry thoroughly, especially between your toes, moisturize, and then slip into a pair of clean socks.

Five-Minute Hand Treatment

Ingredients:

1 tablespoon olive oil

1 tablespoon sugar

Massage this mixture over your fingers and the tops of your hands. Leave on for two minutes, then rinse well with water.

As you see, it doesn't take a lot of money to pamper yourself. Remember this SPA acronym when you get too busy to care for yourself in a special way:

> *Stop*: You need a time-out for yourself once in a while. Take the advice found in Psalm 46:10, "*Be still*, and know that I am God."

> *Pamper*: Give yourself permission to relax your body and renew your spirit by soaking in a bubbly bathtub or lying down while doing a facial. "Perfume and incense bring joy to the heart" (Proverbs 27:9).

> *Appreciate*: Use your quiet time to appreciate what God has done in your life. "Give thanks to the LORD for his unfailing love and his wonderful deeds for men" (Psalm 107:21).

Thought for Rejuvenation

Check off the spa activities you would enjoy:

☐ Facial

☐ Massage

☐ Warm bath

☐ Manicure or pedicure

☐ Napping

☐ Other:

Act of eXpression

Set aside one hour a month for pampering. You can go out for a massage or manicure or stay home for a bubble bath. There are 744 hours in a 31-day month, so you can afford to take one hour and spend it relaxing. When and what will you do this month? Put it on your calendar now.

Day 31

The Splendor of Gray

Do you remember the first day you discovered a gray hair on your head? Did you pluck it or panic? Whether you found your first gray in your thirties, forties, or fifties, that single hair follicle cried out: "You're not as young as you used to be."

Most likely you know a lady who's gone completely gray and looks gorgeous. Her silver hair is sophisticated and attractive, working for her image instead of against it. On the flip side, you've also seen the woman whose gray makes her look, well, frumpy. What makes the difference? How do you know when to accept your grays or when to fight back with Clairol?

If you're beginning to gray, stylists advise you color your hair until you are at least 40 percent gray. Until then, the gray streaks give you an in-between look that ages you instantly. To turn back the clock, try coloring your hair two shades lighter than your natural color (except if you have black hair). At-home hair color is better than ever, so your hair care doesn't have to put a major dent in your wallet. Do keep in mind however that gray hair can be trickier to color because it's usually coarser than your other hair. If you have a hard time making your home hair color stick to the grays, you may need to seek out professional help from a salon.

Here are a few common myths about those silver streaks:

False: You can go gray overnight because of stress.

Fact: A hair shaft can't change color once it has grown in unless it's dyed.

False: If you pull out one gray hair, two more will take its place.

Fact: You will gray follicle by follicle. If you pull out one gray, it will be replaced by one gray.

False: Your hair can return to its natural color after it has gone gray.

Fact: When a hair follicle stops producing pigment, it cannot change back.

By 2030, the U.S. Census Bureau estimates those 65 and older will account for almost 20 percent of the U.S. population (compared to 12.4 percent in 2005).[47] With baby boomers aging, gray is destined to be the new black, especially as people live longer and longer. Also today there are two million Americans in their nineties, and by 2050, that number is estimated to grow to ten million.[48]

American historian and statesman George Bancroft wrote in the 1800s, "By common consent gray hairs are a crown of glory; the only object of respect that can never excite envy."[49] Centuries later that's as true as ever. We respect and admire our elders, but we're not pounding at the door to seek membership.

BEAUTY TIP

Once you've gone mostly gray, choose a short haircut. Long, straggly gray hair will not help you look younger.

Graying and Giving

Infinitely more important than the color of your mane is the integrity of your name. Gray hairs reflect maturity of character and richness of life experience. The wisdom you can pass along to the next generation is priceless. As it says in Titus 2:3-4,

> Likewise, teach the older women to be reverent in the way they live, not to be slanderers or addicted to much wine, but to teach what is good. Then they can train the younger women to love their husbands and children, to be self-controlled and pure, to be busy at home, to be kind, and to be subject to their husbands, so that no one will malign the word of God.

Evelyn, a dear woman at my church, is 100 years old and going strong, a living example of Titus 2:3-4. I spoke with her as she quilted with the Thursday morning church quilting group, her ritual for the past 40 years. She is the matriarch and hero of the group. "Evelyn brings us a new quilt to look at each week," one woman exclaimed. "She's our rock." She teaches the younger women the art of quilting, and by being around her, they also learn the art of living.

Evelyn is passionate about quilting because every quilt is sold to raise money for missionaries. Evelyn is known to stay up late at night to work on her quilts. At 100, she still drives to the grocery store and even picks up other elderly friends who cannot drive anymore. DMV renewed her license until her 103rd birthday.

Her secret to joyful longevity? "Giving is the most important thing in life," said Evelyn, whose accomplishments include raising six kids (three became pastors or missionaries), working on a farm, living through the Depression, visiting shut-ins, and teaching Sunday school for most of her life. "I don't have the gift of speech," she says almost apologetically. But who needs words when her life speaks so loudly? She talks with tears in her eyes about the joy that comes from working for the Lord, trusting Him completely, and fellowshipping with other women (she's been a widow for more than 30 years). She silences the common fears that accompany aging by reading her Bible and seeking the Lord in prayer.

What does she want to do in the future? "I want to continue what I'm doing. I quilt and count the offering every week. I feel young in my heart, but sometimes my legs don't know it." Evelyn has tapped into the fountain of youth by staying active and serving the Lord with everything she's got. Wouldn't it be wonderful to be so independent, needed, and beloved at 100?[50]

Going Green

Beauty doesn't have an expiration date. In fact, you could argue that women become more beautiful as they age. Proverbs 16:31 says, "Gray hair is a crown of splendor; it is attained by a righteous life." In the Bible, age is something to be revered not rejected. True wisdom comes from a history of walking with the Lord, not with the recklessness that often accompanies youth. Job 12:12 puts it this way, "Is not wisdom found among the aged? Does not long life bring understanding?"

With every gray hair, every year spent with Jesus, you are growing in wisdom, grace, and beauty. You're not headed for a junkyard where people with old, clunky parts are put and forgotten. Instead Psalm 92:12-14 paints a much brighter future:

> The righteous will flourish like a palm tree,
> they will grow like a cedar of Lebanon;
> planted in the house of the LORD,
>   they will flourish in the courts of our God.
> They will still bear fruit in old age,
>   they will stay fresh and green.

So as you go gray, may you also remember that you're going green. You will bear fruit. Your life will count. You will have meaningful work. With each day, you are becoming more alive. As you embrace that truth, you will not only feel younger, you'll look younger. Going green isn't just about being good to the environment. It's about the rich quality of life and harvest that can come only with age.

Thought for Rejuvenation

What are your attitudes about aging? Do you have any fears about growing old and going gray?

Act of eXpression

Visit or call someone you admire who is 75 years old or older. Pretend you're a reporter and try to uncover the secret to their success. Ask such questions as:

- What's an average day like for you?

- Tell me about your relationship with God.

- How do you keep in touch with your family?

- What are the highlights of your day?

- Do you exercise regularly?

- How do you keep young at heart?

You Glow, Girl!

"You look fabulous! What's your secret?"
"You haven't aged a bit since our last reunion."
"There's no way you are a grandmother."

How would you like to hear these words spoken about you? I have good news…you will receive compliments like these in the coming weeks and months. People can't help but notice as you give your heart, mind, and body a makeover. If you continue to use the daily prescriptions found in this book, you will be glowing with a love for life, enthusiasm for new adventures, and a healthier, fitter body.

If you ever think you're too old to sizzle, think of my friend who celebrated her fiftieth wedding anniversary this year, and she's got better legs than I do (sad, but true). Or the 78-year-old woman who was leading the dancing at her granddaughter's wedding. Baby boomers and beyond may have aged in years but not in spirit. You don't want to simply retire and fade into the background someday. You yearn to be active and useful, travel, have interesting conversations, and live out the dreams that perhaps have taken a backseat during the childrearing years. You want to feel the passion and energy of your twenties while possessing the wisdom that comes only with age. These wishes can become a reality in your life. Don't believe the cultural lie that your best days are behind you. As a believer in Jesus Christ, your best days are ahead.

Mirror, Mirror on the Wall

I was at SeaWorld with my children, and I had to laugh at something my two-year-old daughter, Noelle, did in the bathroom. As we were leaving, she stopped right in front of the full-length mirror. Looking at herself intently from head to toe, she exclaimed with attitude, "Good!" Not sure of what I'd heard, I asked her, "Noelle, did you just say that you look good?" With a broad smile on her face, she said "Yes."

What a crack up. I'm glad my two-year-old has a positive self-image. So what about you, dear friend? When you look in a full-length mirror and see yourself from head to toe, do you think *good*? Looking and feeling younger is about accepting your appearance, embracing your God-given age, and doing your best to improve your assets. Hear the voice of your heavenly Father as He looks at you, His daughter, and proclaims "Good."

The next time you catch a glimpse of yourself in the mirror, don't forget to smile. You are a luminous work in progress. Beauty has no age limit or expiration date. Aging doesn't mark the end of your journey. It is merely a bridge to many new beginnings God has planned for you. Over the last 31 days, we've looked at your heart, mind, and body. It's been a pleasure to walk alongside of you. Remember…the best is yet to come.

The Top Ten Ways
to Look and Feel Younger

10. Give grace freely to yourself and others.

9. Act like a kid again. Dream, laugh, play, explore.

8. Get eight hours of beauty sleep every night.

7. Avoid wearing too much makeup, elastic waist pants, oversized turtlenecks, and other things that say "old lady."

6. Learn something new every day.

5. Exercise five days a week for 30 minutes or more.

4. Before putting anything in your mouth, ask yourself, *Is this going to hurt or help my body?*

3. Take time out regularly to do what rejuvenates you.

2. Always have something to look forward to.

1. Smile.

Notes

Introduction

1. *The Today Show,* January 18, 2007, http://video.msn.com/?mkt=en-us&brand=msnbc&fg=copy&vid=0598e29a-bd87-4c26-bc81-8e404396129a&from=00.
2. Personal interview with Jane Jaffe, June 24, 2009.
3. Regent University chapel with Zig Ziglar, Spring 1998.

Step 1: Your Personal Rx for the Heart

1. The Free Dictionary, http://www.thefreedictionary.com/fundamental.
2. Dennis Prager, *Happiness Is a Serious Problem* (New York: Regan Books, an imprint of Harper-Collins Publishers, 1998), 5.
3. Rick Warren, *The Purpose Driven Life* (Grand Rapids, MI: Zondervan, 2002), 190.
4. Richard Foster, *The Celebration of Discipline* (New York: HarperCollins, 1978), 17.
5. Ibid., 30.
6. Adapted from Pamela Christian's website, www.blessyourheartcampaign.com/pam.asp.
7. "Healthy Heart Workout Quiz," American Heart Association, www.americanheart.org/presenter.jhtml?identifier=947.
8. Elizabeth George, *A Woman After God's Own Heart* (Eugene, OR: Harvest House Publishers, 1997/2006), 26.
9. Personal conversation with Tami Rosselini, June 21, 2009.
10. Email interview with Vickie Bridges, June 11, 2009.
11. Dan Buettner, interview on *Today Show,* May 16, 2009, http://today.msnbc.msn.com/id/26184891/vp/29876634#30779258.
12. John D. Sutter, "All in the Facebook Family: Older Generations Join Social Networks," CNN.com, April 13, 2009, http://edition.cnn.com/2009/TECH/04/13/social.network.older/index.html.
13. Personal interview with Gracie Rosenberger, Fall 1998.
14. Standing with Hope website, http://www.standingwithhope.com/Gracie.cfm.
15. Charla Krupp, *How Not to Look Old* (New York: Springboard Press, Hachette Book Group USA, 2008), 34.
16. Les Parrott, *The Control Freak* (Carol Stream, IL: Tyndale House Publishers, 2001), 2.
17. Stuart Hample and Eric Marshall, comps., *Children's Letters to God* (New York: Workman Publishing, 1991).

18. Paul S. Joiner, *LifeScripts: Treasured Prayers* (Nashville: Thomas Nelson, n.d.).

19. "The Power of Prayer," from *759 Secrets for Beating Diabetes* (Pleasantville, NY: Reader's Digest Association, 2007).

20. Corrie ten Boom, *Don't Wrestle, Just Nestle* (Old Tappan, NJ: Revell, 1978), 79.

21. Personal phone interview with Mary Tennessen, August 3, 2009.

22. Quoted in Hyrum Smith, *What Matters Most: The Power of Living Your Values* (New York: Simon and Schuster, 2000), 111.

23. Ibid., 66.

24. ExperienceBermuda.com, "What Makes Johnny Wave?" http://www.experiencebermuda.com/sightseeing/friendliest-man.html.

Step 2: Your Personal Rx for the Mind

1. Personal interview with Jane Jaffe, June 24, 2009.

2. Quoted in William Speed Weed, "7 Anti-Aging Tips to Keep Your Brain Young," *Reader's Digest*, n.d., www.rd.com/living-healthy/7-anti-aging-tips-to-keep-your-brain-young/article28203.html.

3. Ibid.

4. Harry Lorayne, *Ageless Memory: Simple Secrets for Keeping Your Brain Young* (New York: Black Dog & Leventhal Publishers, 2007), 56.

5. Personal phone interview with Pam Farrel, July 20, 2009.

6. Personal phone interview with Danna Demetre, July 20, 2009.

7. Weed, "7 Anti-Aging Tips."

8. Personal interview with Debbie Burnett, June 24, 2009.

9. Pam Farrel, *Woman of Confidence: Step into God's Adventure for Your Life* (Eugene, OR: Harvest House Publishers, 2009), 162.

10. Personal phone interview with Kay Laboda, July 15, 2009.

11. "Student Set to Become World's Oldest Graduate," *USA Today*, November 21, 2006, www.usatoday.com/news/offbeat/2006-11-21-lifelong-learner_x.htm.

12. Weed, "7 Anti-Aging Tips."

13. Personal phone interview with Marcia Ramsland, June 11, 2009.

14. Marcia Ramsland, *Simplify Your Life: Get Organized and Stay That Way* (Nashville, TN: W Publishing Group, Thomas Nelson, 2003), 6.

15. Interview with Marcia Ramsland.

16. Personal phone interview with Karen Ehman, September 4, 2009.

17. Marcy Holmes, NP, "Perimenopause Weight Gain—Causes and Solutions," www.womentowomen.com/menopause/menopauseweightgain.aspx.

18. Arlene Pellicane was interviewed at the Crystal Cathedral on May 10, 2009. The interview aired on *The Hour of Power* on May 31, 2009.

19. Pam Farrel, *Fantastic After 40: The Savvy Woman's Guide to Her Best Season of Life* (Eugene, OR: Harvest House Publishers, 2007), 15.

20. Norman Cousins, *Anatomy of an Illness* (New York: W.W. Norton and Company, 1979).

21. Kalia Doner, "5 Habits of Heart-Healthy People," www.remedylife.com/heart/articles/content?cid=346&ctid=2.

22. Daniel J. DeNoon, "Dark Chocolate Is Healthy Chocolate," www.webmd.com/diet/news/20030827/dark-chocolate-is-healthy-chocolate.

23. Interview with Marcia Ramsland.

24. Ibid.

25. Personal phone interview with Carol LeBeau, August 26, 2009.

26. Beverly Buffini, *I Can, I Will, I Believe* (Carlsbad, CA: Olivemount Press, 2003), 109.

27. Martin H. Manser, *The Westminster Collection of Christian Quotations* (Louisville, KY: Westminster John Knox Press, 2001), 49.

Step 3: Your Personal Rx for the Body

1. "Q & A with a Phyllis Diller Plastic Surgeon," Michael Elam, MD, www.cosmeticsurgery.com/articles/archive/an-165/.

2. Jean M. Loftus, MD, *The Smart Woman's Guide to Plastic Surgery* (Chicago: Contemporary Books, 2000), 1.

3. "Menses Overview," www.gynob.com/menses.htm.

4. Interview with Danna Demetre.

5. Colette Bouchez, "Hot Flashes: Open a Window or I'll Scream," www.webmd.com/menopause/guide/hot-flashes-open-window-scream.

6. Pam Farrel, *Fantastic After 40: The Savvy Woman's Guide to Her Best Season of Life* (Eugene, OR: Harvest House Publishers, 2007), 92.

7. Personal phone interview with Karen Ehman, September 4, 2009.

8. Adapted from Karen Ehman's website, http://karenehman.com/home/?page_id=64.

9. Interview with Karen Ehman.

10. Personal phone interview with Danna Demetre, July 20, 2009.

11. Ibid.

12. "100 Ways to Look Younger," *Prevention*, www.prevention.com/100waysyounger/.

13. Morgan Spurlock, *Don't Eat This Book, Fast Food and the Supersizing of America* (New York: G.P. Putnam's Sons, 2005), 60.

14. Ibid., 19.

15. Personal phone interview with Chelle Stafford, February 27, 2009.

16. Ibid.

17. Spurlock, *Don't Eat This Book*, 151.

18. Richard Foster, *The Celebration of Discipline* (New York: HarperCollins, 1978), 55.

19. "Water: The Elixir of Life," www.parentingweekly.com/pregnancy/breathingspace/vol38/pregnancy_health_fitness.asp.

20. "Help for Soda Lovers," www.webmd.com/food-recipes/features/help-soda-lovers.

21. Interview with Danna Demetre.

22. Personal interview with my mom, Ann Kho, January 15, 2009.

23. *2008 Physical Activity Guidelines for Americans*, U.S. Department of Health and Human Services, www.health.gov/paguidelines/guidelines/default.aspx.

24. Beth Howard, "In Your Dreams: How to Sleep Better, Longer, Easier and Reap More of the Health Benefits of Getting Enough Rest," *Healthy Living*, Summer 2009, www.remedylife.com/general/articles/content?cid=1919&ctid=2.

25. Personal interview with Michelle Anderson, November 9, 2007.

26. Howard, "In Your Dreams."

27. Kalia Doner, "5 Habits of Heart-Healthy People," *Remedy*, August 2006, www.remedylife.com/heart/articles/content?cid=346&ctid=2.

28. Bill and Pam Farrel, *Red Hot Monogamy: Making Your Marriage Sizzle* (Eugene, OR: Harvest House Publishers, 2006), 157.

29. Ed Wheat, MD, *Intended for Pleasure: Sex Techniques and Sexual Fulfillment in Christian Marriage* (Grand Rapids, MI: Revell, 1977), 216.

30. Personal phone interview with Pam Farrel, July 20, 2009.

31. Wheat, *Intended for Pleasure,* 128.

32. Interview with Pam Farrel.

33. "Get My Teeth" joke, http://blog.seniors-site.com/get-my-teeth-joke.

34. Personal phone interview with Kathy Martin, August 27, 2009.

35. Patsy Clairmont, "Word of the Month," September 2009, www.patsyclairmont.com/word .html.

36. Women of Faith conference, September 5, 2008, Anaheim, CA.

37. Personal interview with Jane Jaffe, June 24, 2009.

38. John and Stasi Eldredge, *Captivating: Unveiling the Mystery of a Woman's Soul* (Nashville, TN: Thomas Nelson Publishers, 2007), 6.

39. http://thinkexist.com/quotation/beauty_is_how_you_feel_inside-and_it_reflects_in/220285 .html.

40. Ken Gire, *Windows of the Soul* (Grand Rapids, MI: Zondervan, 1996), 18.

41. http://thinkexist.com/quotation/every_time_you_smile_at_someone-it_is_an_action/215120 .html.

42. Personal phone interview with Thelma Wells, July 16, 2009.

43. Doris J. Day, MD, *Forget the Facelift: Dr. Day Turns Back the Clock with a Revolutionary Program for Ageless Skin* (New York: Penguin Group, 2005), 75.

44. Ibid., 91.

45. American Massage Therapy Association website, www.amtamassage.org/news/MTIndustry FactSheet.html#6.

46. Colette Bouchez, "Spas: The Risks and Benefits," www.webmd.com/skin-problems-and-treat ments/features/spas-the-risks-and-benefits.

47. J. Walker Smith and Ann Clurman, *Generation Ageless: How Baby Boomers Are Changing the Way We Live Today and They're Just Getting Started* (New York: HarperCollins Publishers, 2007), 8.

48. *The Today Show,* October 27, 2008, http://today.msnbc.msn.com/id/26184891/vp/29876634 #27399360.

49. www.brainyquote.com/quotes/authors/g/george_bancroft.html.

50. Personal interview with Evelyn Birdwell and quilting group at San Diego First Assembly of God, August 27, 2009.

About Arlene Pellicane

Before becoming a stay-at-home mom, Arlene worked as the associate producer for *Turning Point Television* with Dr. David Jeremiah as well as a features producer for *The 700 Club*. From her experience of five pregnancies in five years (including two miscarriages), Arlene developed *Losing Weight After Baby: 31 Days to a New You*, an audio book to encourage and motivate moms.

Arlene has appeared as a guest on *The Hour of Power* and *The 700 Club*. An energetic communicator, she shares compelling and heartwarming stories to guide her audiences to positive life-change. She loves speaking at seminars, moms groups, special events, and retreats.

Arlene received her BA in intercultural studies from Biola University and her masters in journalism from Regent University. In addition to writing during her young children's naptimes, Arlene enjoys traveling, bargain hunting, and eating her husband's home-made kettle corn. Arlene and her husband, James, live in Southern California with their three children Ethan, Noelle, and Lucy.

www.ArlenePellicane.com

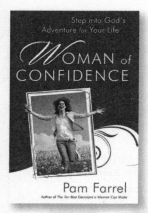

Woman of Confidence
Step into God's Adventure for Your Life
Pam Farrel

Popular speaker and relationship specialist Pam Farrel, coauthor of *Men Are Like Waffles, Women Are Like Spaghetti,* helps you discover how to develop the confidence you need to walk into your hopes, dreams, and aspirations. The strongest, most confident women know God and look at life from His point of view.

With plenty of biblical examples and practical insights, along with a dash of humor, Farrel reveals that nothing is more vital to your self-confidence than your confidence in God.

Each chapter of *Woman of Confidence* contains:

- *Winning Words*—Scripture to help you feel empowered and overcome your fears
- *Winning Wisdom*—Tools you can use to achieve your dreams
- *Winner's Circle*—Inspirational nuggets you can post for encouragement and motivation
- *Winning Ways*—Accountability partner exercises and questions perfect for prayer partners, girlfriends, or small groups

Great for women's groups or for individual encouragement, *Woman of Confidence* helps you understand that mustering up enough *self*-confidence is not the answer. Your ability to achieve, to move through life with courage and boldness, rests instead on the character, power, and strength of God.

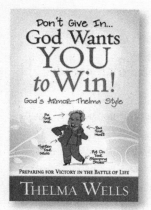

Don't Give In…God Wants You to Win!
Preparing for Victory in the Battle of Life
Thelma Wells

Popular author and conference speaker Thelma Wells will inspire you to fight the good fight of faith and win the raging wars that you battle each day as the enemy tries to steal your joy, kill your hopes and dreams, and destroy your life. In her personable and enthusiastic style, Wells helps you understand:

- what spiritual warfare is
- why you fight
- who you are fighting
- how to dress for the war
- how to win the war
- who ultimately is in control of the fight

Don't Give In…God Wants You to Win! will cause you to understand that the battles you fight are really not yours. Those battles belong to the God of "Peace, be still," who will give you the strategies and courage you need to resist Satan's tricks.

Wells writes for anyone fighting battles over family, relationships, finances, health, broken dreams, disappointments, and just the dailyness of life that can cause so much distress and hurt. Through instruction from God's Word and stories of modern-day as well as biblical people, Wells shows how to relinquish those troubles to the only Person who can guarantee winning strategies for life.

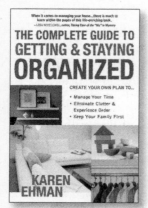

The Complete Guide to Getting and Staying Organized
Karen Ehman

The key to good organization is not a one-size-fits-all method. It is a unique plan that considers personality type, lifestyle, income level, and family schedule. Author and speaker Karen Ehman believes that with her simple step-by-step process you can recognize your personal style of managing your household successfully and develop a unique plan that gives you the freedom to:

- manage your time wisely
- declutter and organize your home
- plan menus, shop more efficiently, and become more comfortable and creative in the kitchen
- get your children involved in pursuing an ordered life and home
- avoid the trap of overcommitment
- use practical tools to assist in organization

Getting and staying organized means more time for the important things in family life—concentrating on cultivating a close, personal relationship with the Creator, drawing His Word into every aspect of living, and ultimately tying your children's heartstrings to God.

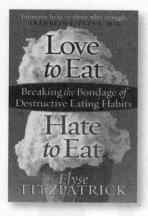

Love to Eat, Hate to Eat
Breaking the Bondage of Destructive Eating Habits
Elyse Fitzpatrick

More than 80 percent of all Americans have been on a diet at some point in their lives. Low fat, low carb, high protein—you name it—they've tried it. Isn't there a better way to break the cycle in the battle of the bulge?

After years of futile dieting, we all know there's more to weight control than what we eat. Having discovered the power that food has over our lives, counselor Elyse Fitzpatrick, author of *Overcoming Fear, Worry, and Anxiety*, helps us:

- identify destructive eating habits
- break the vicious cycle of emotional eating
- develop a flexible plan suited to unique situations

God knows everything about us…where we've been and where we're going. Because He knows us so well, He can deeply transform us, giving us the contentment we long for.

To learn more about other Harvest House books
or to read sample chapters, log on to our website:

www.harvesthousepublishers.com

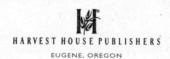

HARVEST HOUSE PUBLISHERS
EUGENE, OREGON